Join the legions of readers who have transformed their bodies, minds, and lives for good, with Joe Manganiello—the man director Steven Soderbergh dubbed "WALKING CGI." The question is: HOW BAD DO YOU WANT IT?

PRAISE FOR EVOLUTION

"This isn't a jock talking about building muscles, it's a man encouraging people to free themselves of limits as he did, to value ambition, hustle, and a healthy mind-set."

—*People*

"A comprehensive yet straightforward and effective road-map to better health and fitness, not to mention a killer physique—the kind that may just have people wondering if you're not a fitness expert yourself. After reading *Evolution*, you will be."

—Shawn Perine, editor-in-chief of *Muscle & Fitness*

"Joe Manganiello's picture is next to the definition of 'fitness' in *Webster's Dictionary*. He is one of the most creative and motivated people I know. You'll be inspired. And if that's not enough of a reason, a free lap dance comes with every book!"

—Channing Tatum, star of the *Magic Mike* films and *People*'s 2012 Sexiest Man Alive

"Joe lives it twenty-four/seven. I've been training for more than forty years, and a body like that involves two factors: incredible work ethic and inhuman discipline. Joe has those along with diet dialed to perfection. As they say, the proof is in the pudding."

—2015 WWE Hall of Fame inductee "Big Sexy" Kevin Nash

"This book will give you real results. Using simple, easy-to-do routines and dietary recommendations . . . I was able to put on ten pounds of muscle in one month. Listen to Joe—he won't let you down!"

—Matt Bomer, 2015 Golden Globes winner
for *The Normal Heart*

"[Joe] and his trainer approached me and we started talking work ethic and discipline as far as health and nutrition were concerned . . . there was a mutual understanding of hard work and dedication and what it takes for those two aspects to pay off. Two years have passed, and I can honestly say that I am inspired and fortunate—Joe has been a positive force in my life! Turn-up!"

—Marcedes Lewis, All-Pro NFL Jacksonville Jaguars tight end

"Manganiello rewrites the book on getting ripped."

—*Daily News*

"If you want to know whether or not Joe Manganiello understands the mechanics of health and fitness, JUST LOOK AT HIM. Okay, stop staring. Now you're being creepy."

—Chris Hardwick, host of AMC's *Talking Dead* and BBC America's *The Nerdist*

"While filming in Atlanta, Joe and I lifted regularly and hard. He showed me some of his routines and let me in on a few secrets. When I got home my wife put out BIG-TIME! Joe's book is a must-have for anyone who likes getting laid!"

—Max Martini, star of Warner Brothers' *Pacific Rim*

"A day after working out with Joe Manganiello feels like the morning after going twelve rounds with Tyson. This is Hollywood's hardest workout."

—Dan Jones, editor-at-large for *Men's Health* UK

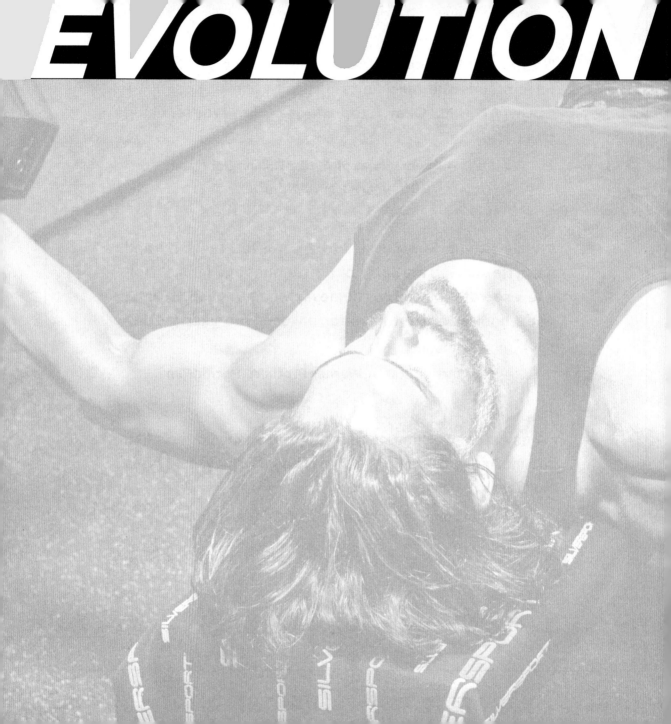

JOE MANGANIELLO

WORKOUTS DESIGNED BY RON MATHEWS

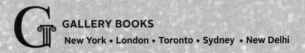

GALLERY BOOKS

New York • London • Toronto • Sydney • New Delhi

G

Gallery Books
An Imprint of Simon & Schuster, Inc.
1230 Avenue of the Americas
New York, NY 10020

First Gallery Books trade paperback edition October 2015

GALLERY BOOKS and colophon are registered trademarks of Simon & Schuster, Inc.

For information about special discounts for bulk purchases, please contact Simon & Schuster Special Sales at 1-866-506-1949 or business@simonandschuster.com.

The Simon & Schuster Speakers Bureau can bring authors to your live event. For more information or to book an event, contact the Simon & Schuster Speakers Bureau at 1-866-248-3049 or visit our website at www.simonspeakers.com.

Interior design by Jaime Putorti

Top left photo on p. xi courtesy of Freyvogel Photography
All other photography by Patrik Giardino
Styling by Caprice Gray
Cover design by Bau-Da Design

Manufactured in the United States of America

10 9 8 7 6 5 4 3 2 1

Library of Congress Cataloging-in-Publication Data is available for the hardcover edition.

ISBN 978-1-4767-1670-1
ISBN 978-1-4767-1671-8 (pbk)
ISBN 978-1-4767-1672-5 (ebook)

CONTENTS

Back

Legs

Triceps

FOREWORD

BY ARNOLD SCHWARZENEGGER

This year, I lost someone very dear to me, someone who shaped my life. Joe Weider passed away in March and I lost a father figure and a mentor. At the same time, the world lost one of the greatest advocates of fitness, the godfather of bodybuilding.

In case you don't know, it was Joe Weider who inspired me with his magazines to embrace bodybuilding as the blueprint to all of my dreams, and it was Joe Weider who brought me to America so I could make those dreams come true. It was Joe Weider who started the fitness crusade that I've been on for more than four decades.

When we sat down to plan his memorial, I wanted to honor his memory and show his tremendous impact on the world. It was a no-brainer to invite bodybuilding legends like Franco Columbu and Lou Ferrigno to speak.

But I also wanted someone to represent the next generation of action stars and lifters, to truly show Joe Weider's impact.

In the beginning of my career, when I started promoting fitness, gyms were dungeons, hidden away from the general population. People spoke about weight training in whispers—as if those of us who did it were freaks. Now, there are gyms everywhere you look and doctors recommend weight training.

When I started looking for a younger speaker who would be able to understand Joe Weider's legacy and also serve as a new flag bearer for the fitness crusade, it was obvious.

I called my friend Joe Manganiello.

"Joe, the Joe Weider memorial is this weekend, and I'd like you to speak about what he meant to you."

He sounded taken aback. "Are you sure, Arnold? That room will be filled with the bodybuilding greats. I'm not sure I've made it to the level where I should be speaking on that stage."

I said, "See you Sunday."

I had no question about whether Joe belonged on the stage.

When we worked on our film *Sabotage* together, I immediately noticed Joe's passion for health and fitness. Well, that isn't true. First I noticed his huge arms and cannonball delts.

We ate lunch together almost every day, and I found out we had a lot in common. Joe was a construction worker who worked in masonry to get by while he waited for his big break. And I was a construction worker who started a bricklaying business with my best friend Franco to get by when bodybuilding didn't pay.

So at least if all else fails, we know that we could start a fantastic construction company together.

The more we talked, I couldn't shake the feeling that Joe is perfect to keep fighting the fitness crusade Joe Weider started and I've continued for all these years. This is someone who truly believes in fitness, not someone who crash-diets because his contract says he has to look great with his shirt off. He'd still have those biceps if he never got his break and was laying bricks. Most importantly, he believes in old-fashioned hard work above everything else. Everyone can see how this has paid off in his career—Joe's body is a costar in his film and TV work because of the work he does, and he has become a sex symbol and an inspiration for men and women.

We talked constantly about our shared belief that there is no shortcut to health and fitness. We both firmly believe that any time you waste looking for a shortcut or a magic pill is time that you could have spent working your ass off.

One day, Joe told me that he wanted to write this book. He was inspired by my *Encyclopedia of Modern Bodybuilding* when he was young and he wanted to inspire the next generation.

I couldn't have been happier.

This book is meant as a wake-up call. It's an alarm that is going off to tell you it's time to stop waiting. It's time to stop complaining. It's time to start your Evolution and be the best version of yourself.

Not tomorrow. Now.

It's not easy to define the "best version of yourself." So let's put it this way.

Each night, go to bed as the best version of yourself . . . so far.

Each morning, wake up with a plan to end the day as a new, better version.

I have always called this "staying hungry." Joe calls it *Evolution*.

No matter what you call it, it is the path to a happy and healthy life.

This book does not promise any magic spells or gimmicks. That's why I love it. But if you start reading today, you will be better tomorrow. And the next day. And the day after that.

That Sunday, as Joe stood at the podium at the Weider memorial and told the crowd how proud he was that he had gone from being the little boy dreaming while he read the Weider magazines to being the man on the cover of the most widely read fitness and bodybuilding magazine in the world inspiring the next generation, I knew I'd made the right choice.

You've made it, Joe.

Everybody else, pay attention.

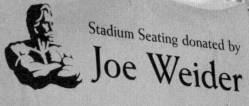

EVOLUTION

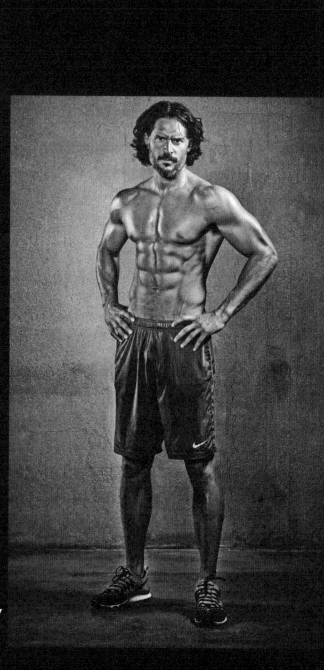

Me then

Me now

INTRODUCTION

When that first picture was taken, if you could have sat me down and showed me the second picture and told the little me where my life would wind up, I never would have believed you in a million years.

Hell, there are pictures of me from fifteen years ago where I struggle to see the resemblance to the guy on-screen in *True Blood* and *Magic Mike*.

Looking at the kid in the first picture takes me back to a place and time where the dreams of looking like the action movie stars and comic book heroes that I grew up idolizing were merely that: *dreams*. In fact, I think the word "dream" is even a bit too presumptive, because there is no way I could have possibly cooked up any of this in my mind.

If you told scrawny me that one day I would appear on the cover of just about every major fitness and bodybuilding magazine in the world and then be asked to write a cutting-edge book of modern fitness, I would have looked at you cross-eyed. Then if you told me that I would be asked by my childhood idol, Arnold Schwarzenegger, to speak on behalf of my generation at the memorial service of bodybuilding godfather Joe Weider, alongside people like Lou Ferrigno, I would have gotten up and walked away. No one in his right mind would have ever imagined that the skinny kid you see in that picture would end up seated at the head table with the Hulk and the Terminator, leading the charge to improve the future of fitness.

Yet here we are.

That picture is meant to spark the ignition of change, so that the word can be spread: *everyone* possesses the capability to look the way he or she wants.

I believe the culture we live in has some serious problems in terms of health and fitness. This book is my rallying cry, my St. Crispin's Day speech. I'm putting together an army, a force for cultural change, and *I want you*! It's time to stop with the "Nice try!" pats on the back. I'm going to tell you like it is, say what needs to be said, and then draw a line in the sand. You can determine which side you're going to stand on.

I don't make my living in fitness, and I don't need to sell you anything but the truth. I've read those celebrity workouts and diets that come at you with the quick fixes, a magical diet, or some lost secret that they guarantee will give you "Razor Sharp Abs!" or whatever other unrealistic promises you might see in a magazine. I've appeared on the covers of those magazines and been featured in their articles and can tell you one thing: while the content is great, the programs are incomplete. The solutions don't show the entire story: the mental or the physical. Or the inevitable hurdles you will encounter as you transform your body and mind.

That's not to knock all of those magazines. Some of them are run by great fitness minds and are full of fantastic information. They are a piece of the puzzle. But if you really want to look like those guys in the magazines, then the advice you're being offered by the mainstream is just scratching the surface. It's deeper than how many reps you need to do on the bench press to build your pectoral muscles or the number of curls it takes to actually make your biceps stretch your shirtsleeves.

It's about teaching you what buttons to push and how to push them harder and more consistently than anyone has ever showed you before.

EVOLUTION IS REBIRTH

I know this because I used to push all the wrong buttons, at all the wrong times, in all the wrong ways. I was brought down by previous failures and preconceived notions about what I could become. I unknowingly set myself up to fail time after time, and I began to believe I just wasn't born to be built a certain way. While growing up in Mt. Lebanon, Pennsylvania, there was even a time when I was picked on and bullied by the older kids at school. What people see today isn't representative of what I had to go through in order to learn to fight back and rise above the hurdles and barriers of life. I had to learn how to overcome some massive difficulties every step of the way.

When it came to fitness, I was a young man who coasted on his potential and who was no stranger to rock bottom. For years, I struggled to get in shape and live a healthy lifestyle. As an adult, those same struggles galvanized my resolve to search out the best ways to become successful and build a body that represented who I truly was and what I could achieve. My story isn't about genetic luck or random chance. Maybe the only thing I can say I did right was that I never gave up. I fought tirelessly and searched for techniques, mentors, and methods to become better. For the time it takes to read and implement this book, I'm going to save you a lot of my struggle by giving you all the answers.

The only difference between us, as I see it, is that I have figured out the "secrets" that actually work.

Secret 1: There are no secrets.

EVOLUTION IS A MIND-SET

Evolution starts once you can grasp and accept the infinite possibilities and agree to never cut corners or make excuses. A lot of people want to assume that I didn't have to work to become what I am. That it was all about genetics and a body that was given to me—not earned. I think it's because they can't fathom putting in the work themselves. They want to believe there is a golden ticket that exists for certain people, and maybe there is, but I sure as hell didn't get it!

It doesn't matter if you've been pushing yourself in the gym for years or have avoided it entirely out of fear. I can say with the utmost confidence that these techniques will actually work for you.

EVOLUTION IS NOT A QUICK FIX

Changes *can* happen fast, but understand that this book goes much deeper than merely telling you which exercises to perform and the right foods to eat. This program is all-encompassing: mental, physical, and spiritual. What good is teaching you the physical side if you're not supplied with the mind-set you need to push past the barriers and process the frustration that typically holds people back? I want this to be the book that changes your life. I'm living proof that it can, because what's contained here completely transformed mine.

EVOLUTION IS FAITH

One of the best things I've ever had going for me is that I never do anything half-assed. In more than a few aspects of my life, I've sometimes paid a heavy price for being that way. But in terms of fitness, I can say that what I have put in, I've gotten back tenfold. When I trust my gut and go at a goal with 110 percent effort, and *act as if* I'm 110 percent sure that what I'm doing is going to work—that's when the incredible happens.

I recommend that you do the same here. If you've picked up this book, there's obviously something that you think you're missing. If you're capable of taking direction and pushing yourself like you've never done before, then I can say with complete confidence that you are going to change!

Much in the way that Arnold Schwarzenegger wrote the *Encyclopedia of Modern Bodybuilding* in 1987, *Evolution* is meant to stand on its shoulders as the next chapter. I'm using techniques that have been long forgotten and others that have been completely overlooked. This is the sum total of what we know and how far we've come.

ARE YOU READY TO EVOLVE?

Your transformation begins the moment you turn the page.

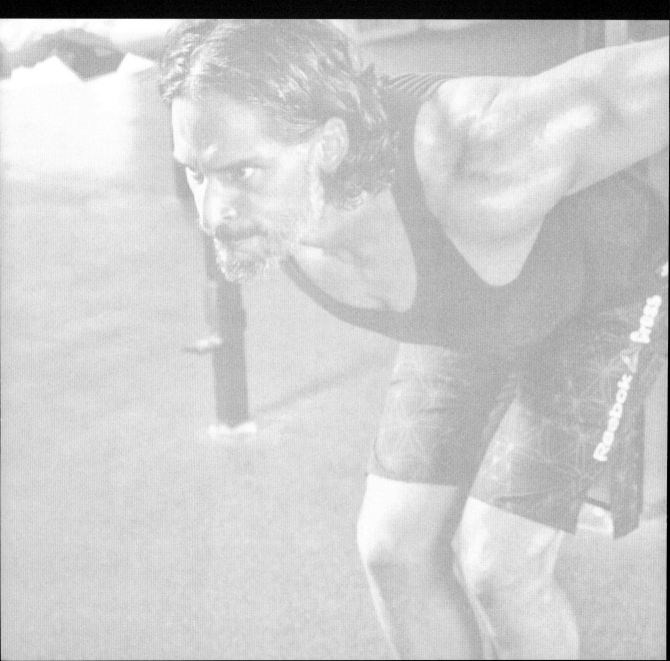

CHAPTER 1

Failure
Is the
Foundation
of
Success

We live in a society that is headed in a frightening direction. It is rapidly becoming a culture that shields our fragile egos from failure. The result is a society of people who applaud potential instead of results, and a mentality of "good enough" rather than "better than ever."

Our hypersensitive society has created a mentality that can't handle failure. Whether you're first or last, we preach "Good try!" instead of "Work harder." We do it with everything, and we do it in the worst ways possible, such as with our health. We coddle ourselves, and it's the reason why so many people think it's okay to be overweight and out of shape. Or why so many have rationalized their inability to exercise and eat in a healthy way. You fail once and then tell yourself that something better isn't a possibility.

The reality? You've been taught to quit at failure. You don't smell success, because there's no incentive to push forward. There's no hurt, pain, or disappointment when you fall short. For you to evolve, that must all change.

The problem is apparent everywhere. Look no further than today's youth. Children play sports games where goals aren't counted and everyone gets a trophy at the end. I'm all for providing a nurturing environment for children to grow up in. Heck, almost all of the charity organizations I work with are designed to provide better lives for kids. But people need to be pushed—both externally and internally. That internal fire can never burn without some fuel, and that fuel can come in the form of disappointment, embarrassment, and even jealously. The poison, no doubt, is in the dose, as these traits are incredibly corrosive if held on to for extended periods of time, but if you can learn to convert them into positive actions, they can help you tremendously.

I benefitted from failure. I needed to feel it. I needed to sit in it. I needed to know what losing felt like, and I needed to get angry about it and never want to feel that way again. Without it, I would have been robbed of the lifeblood that has propelled me all these years later. It would have eliminated my opportunity to stand taller.

I hate failing, and, even worse, I hate admitting it. But at night, I can look at myself in the mirror and know that every time I did fail, it was the best thing for me. I got back up, devised a better plan of action, and went back with fire in my stomach for those who doubted me when I told them what I wanted to achieve, changes I desired to make, and who I wanted to become.

I issue that same challenge to you. I want you to look at your failures, embrace them, and immerse yourself in them. Then I want you to use that pain as fuel and set up this one seemingly simple goal: What can you change in a year?

I'm going to need you to accept nothing less than your best effort. You owe it to yourself to know, once and for all, how far you can go. I want you to look in that mirror and love what you see, inside and out. I want you to feel like you've earned your sleep at night.

All I ask is that you believe that what I'm telling you has worked for me and to do the footwork.

What do you see when you look at yourself?

It's an honest question that I asked myself years ago. What you see now when you look at me did not occur by accident, and it wasn't easy. My "instant" success was a twenty-year journey, and I want the path I took to inspire in you the confidence to rise up after you're kicked in the face. Because as you're about to learn, the most impressive people in the world are the ones who suffered from failure and learned how to respond.

After I played Flash Thompson in the movie *Spider-Man* in 2002, I ended up not acting for *four* years. How does this happen? The ins and outs of my fall from acting boil down to a vicious cycle caused by my drinking too much, smoking too much, and acting like I had won the lifetime lottery, because I'd had a role in a big movie. It began a downward spiral that resulted in my getting dumped off of my own personal elevator to hell, at the bottom floor.

One of my professors at the Carnegie Mellon University School of Drama, Victoria Santa Cruz, used to say, "The moment you say 'I did it!' is the moment the devil walks in the door," and that's exactly what happened to me.

I spent several years in a blur and for the most part was unhireable. I had immense trouble finding the will to motivate myself to do simple things such as leave the house, let alone train the way I wanted. I began to accept that most likely acting wasn't going to happen for me; that I had gotten into the wrong profession out of ego, had burned too many bridges and made a mistake. My mind spun all day, consumed by the question "What if?" *What if* I could somehow get out of my own way long enough to make a change? And unbelievably, through a series of bizarre events—and, looking back, perhaps divine intervention—I found it within myself to begin the process of cleaning up my life.

Through a friend of a friend, I was introduced to this professional hockey player: an NHL enforcer who had been suspended by the league multiple times. We became instant buddies. He mentioned that he needed a sparring partner to help him get back in shape and make his push to return to the league. We bonded over our similar struggles, and little did I know it, his comeback would mirror my own, in ways that I could have never imagined.

I had never really boxed before in any structured way, but I had absolutely nothing else going on for me, so I said yes.

We started boxing training three times a week. It was a habit that helped me put an end to my other vice: chain-smoking. We'd get in the gym at six o'clock in the evening. I'd make sure I wouldn't smoke beforehand, and then afterward, I'd eat, shower, and go straight to bed—before the urge to smoke could overtake me. That good habit led to other good habits, and just like that, my entire mind-set began changing.

I was no longer seeing what I could get away with; I was seeing what I could *do*.

FINDING REDEMPTION

Eventually my friend went back to hockey, and I was left with an empty bank account, not having worked as an actor in four years. I now faced the overwhelming question of what to do with the rest of my life. I had always loved the book *The Fountainhead* by Ayn Rand, which is loosely based on the life and personality of the famous architect Frank Lloyd Wright. At one point in the story, the protagonist's personal life and career as an architect completely implode. He is forced to close his office, and he decides to take a job breaking rocks all day at a quarry. I was always confused by and in total awe of that gesture. The fact that this highly trained, brilliant architect would lower himself and take an entry-level manual-labor job had perplexed me for years. Why would he do that? I decided to find out for myself.

I took a job at a masonry company working long days, shoveling sand and gravel from seven in the morning until four in the afternoon.

In my mind, my acting career was over. No one would return my phone calls, and I'd been rejected by every agent and manager in town. There was something about driving the truck in the morning, picking up my orders, and shutting off my brain and shoveling for hours.

During that first week, I thought I was going to die. I couldn't see how I was going to make it through. My back hurt, my legs and shoulders hurt, and I started waking up with a throbbing headache every morning. I took Advil and drank plenty of fluids, but nothing would get rid of that headache—that is, until I started breaking a sweat by shoveling in the 90-degree Los Angeles heat each morning. I was like a junkie or an alcoholic with the DTs, shaking violently until I got my morning fix. It was as if my body and soul were screaming at me, "You need this!" I showed up day after day for work on that truck and within weeks my body started changing drastically. It was as though for my entire life, there had been a genetic barrier inside me that was stopping me from filling out physically and packing on muscle, but my daily construction workouts removed it completely.

At this point, I was almost three years off of drinking and two years removed from smoking. I started getting serious about my diet and made it my business to go to the gym after those long days working construction. I was twenty-eight years old, and I wanted to see how much I could fill out. I wanted to know what it would be like to be *big*.

I took that job in construction because I needed to pay my bills, but the act of humbling myself and accepting who I was and where I was changed my life. For the first time in a long time, I started to grow. Working that difficult job epitomized the anti-ego mentality that I needed to begin really succeeding. Slowly but surely, I began to understand why the hero in *The Fountainhead* took the job at the quarry. The monotonous, repetitive physical labor was a cleanse of sorts for my head and my soul. I was alone in my bubble every day finding out exactly what I was made of. I was taking inventory and digesting everything I had been through. I still thought my dream of an acting career was over, but in the meantime, I was going to become the greatest shoveler, cement mixer, and jackhammer operator of all time.

Looking back, that humbling experience is what turned me into the man I am today, in just about every way.

With the addition of those postconstruction gym sessions, I began pushing my life back into alignment. I didn't just train after work; I hit the gym like an animal. I pushed myself to the point where the people around me were borderline frightened. I was a man on a mission.

WHY POTENTIAL SUCKS

How hard have you pushed yourself?

That's the question I want you to ask. Got your answer? Good, 'cause now it's time for a little love.

Tough love.

Most guys don't realize that the hard work they put in isn't enough. They look around and wonder why everyone else has success. They want to know why they can't catch a break. You know why it doesn't happen for them? It's because those who reap the benefits of life don't wait for breaks to happen; they *make* them happen. It's an aggressive approach to life and an endless pursuit that will lead to what you want. The best don't see a locked door and walk away in another direction. They wind up and kick the damn thing down! Or better yet, they smash through the brick wall next to the door, because they can.

During my fall, I had become okay with being comfortable. Comfortable with being average and less than I wanted. Comfortable with not rising up or pushing back when I was knocked down and not being a little tougher. As a result, I settled for less.

Those who truly evolve are the ones who leap off of life's cliffs. Their world is not one of haves and have-nots, and it's not one of potential. It's one of hustle, ambition, and endless determination.

My wish for you is to have that magic moment like I did in which you fully take responsibility and eliminate your excuses.

I'm not passing judgment here. I'm merely letting you know what it took for me to make the most out of all my opportunities and what it will take for you to get more than you think is possible.

Don't accept yourself as a finished product. *Ever*. We all have weaknesses. And those weaknesses don't mean that you're weak. It means that you have so much more you can accomplish.

What would have happened if Michael Jordan quit when his game wasn't good enough for him to make his varsity basketball team?

What if Arnold Schwarzenegger had listened to all the naysayers in his tiny little village in Austria on his way to becoming the world's greatest bodybuilder? Or action star? Or governor?

What if Steve Jobs had quit after Apple failed and was being crushed by the PC world?

Those who work on their weaknesses, shortcomings, and/or failures are destined to become great. Those who don't, fall behind.

GREAT PEOPLE WHO OVERCAME SETBACKS AND FAILURES

Arnold Schwarzenegger	Walt Disney	Jerry Seinfeld
Michael Jordan	Albert Einstein	Steven Spielberg
Steve Jobs	Oprah Winfrey	J. K. Rowling
Henry Ford	Thomas Edison	the Beatles
	Harrison Ford	

Acceptance is an inner state of humility achieved only after a period of grueling and thorough hard work. Falling flat on your face and then getting up for more.

I shudder to think of the way my life could have gone if I had talked myself out of auditioning for the Carnegie Mellon University School of Drama, due to the fact that I didn't have the money to afford the tuition, even if I was accepted. In fact, it would have been even easier for me to give up after I did muster up the courage to audition right out of high school—only to be subsequently rejected.

They told me "no." I had failed . . . but I knew that I could do better. So I came up with a plan.

I decided to attend the University of Pittsburgh because (A) I could afford the in-state tuition, (B) they had a liberal arts theatre studies program, and (C) the campus was within walking distance to Carnegie Mellon.

It was time to go to work.

That first semester, I took every acting class I could fit into my schedule. It got to the point where my guidance counselor pulled me aside and suggested that I ease up, due to the fact that I would use up all of my theatre courses in my first two years . . . but I never had any idea of being there past the first.

I auditioned for every play I could at Pitt and wound up being cast in lead roles in several of them, much to the chagrin of some of the graduate students.

I answered every possible casting notice I could find in the paper. I rode endless subways and bus transfers to auditions and shoots for the most amateur, local, nonpaying, crazy video jobs you could possibly imagine, just so I could get in front of a camera.

I took classes studying all of the classic plays and signed up for film philosophy classes.

I volunteered for photo shoots with up-and-coming photographers in return for free headshots.

All the while, I was developing new audition monologues that I would practice performing for the kids who lived down the hall from me in my dorm.

After being rejected by CMU, I spent every single moment of that year making myself better and finding out how much I could change and grow. If I was going to be rejected a second time after that year, then I needed to be able to look back and know that I did everything I possibly could. That was the only way that I knew of that I could possibly walk away from my dream.

That year flew by, and one fateful Saturday morning in early February, I walked across Forbes Avenue from Pitt to CMU and tried out again. I didn't apply to any other schools and I never had a backup plan. That was it. There was no "Plan B."

I got in.

That year, I was one of only seventeen actors accepted out of eight hundred, and upon learning of my financial situation, the head of CMU's acting department found a 75 percent scholarship for me to attend.

Looking back at my life, it was the obstacles, the shortcomings, and the failures that forced me to fight harder, to reach inside and pull something truly extraordinary out of myself that I didn't even know existed. My failure was essential to my growth, because every time I failed, I learned that it was because I did not fight as hard as *humanly possible.*

Notice I didn't say "fight my hardest." There are a lot of people who try as hard as they can. But their ceilings and limitations are *perceived* barriers that restrict what they can achieve. We don't know what we can really do until we push past the farthest point we've ever been and go where we've never gone before. There is a place beyond the conscious perception of what is achievable and *that* is where real success occurs.

After years of failure, I learned that there was another gear some-where inside of me, and oftentimes it took failing to find the upshift. I began to believe that if, given enough time, and if I followed an intelligent and disciplined plan, I could change so drastically that you wouldn't even recognize me. I had learned to evolve.

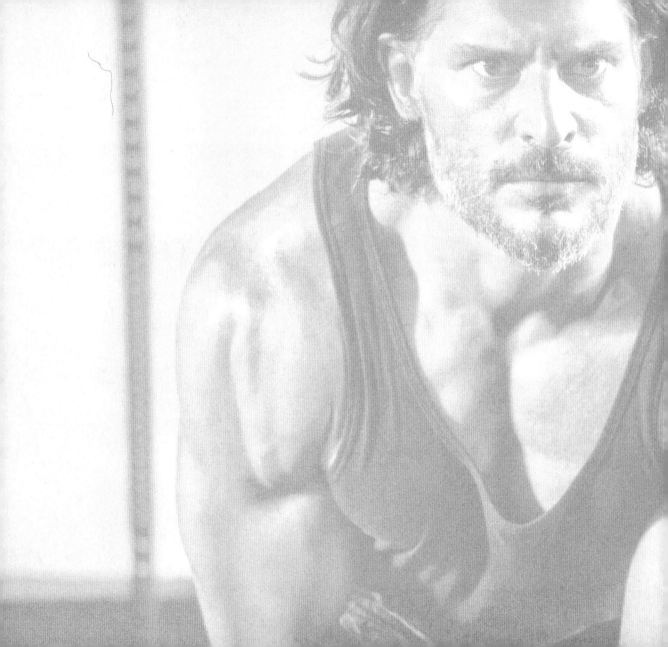

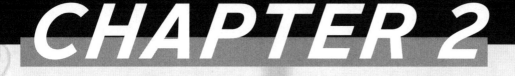

CHAPTER 2

3:59,
the Number That Will
Change Your Life

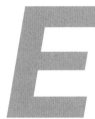**E**very time you have a doubt about what I tell you in this book, I want you to think of Roger Bannister.

For those of you who don't know the story of Bannister, he was a distinguished English neurologist and Olympic runner in the 1950s. If you look in the record books, you'll be hard-pressed to find Bannister's name anywhere—with one exception. He was the first man to run a sub-four-minute mile.

While this might not seem like much now, breaking this barrier was actually once considered *impossible*. The mile has existed since ancient Roman times. It is a unit of length equivalent to 5,280 feet (1,760 yards, or about 1,609 meters), originally used by the Roman army to signify the length of one thousand paces of a Roman legion, with each pace equaling two steps. For thousands of years, no one— not one single person—could eclipse the four-minute mark. For that reason, sportswriters and even physicists postulated that human evolution had certain limits and that running a mile in less than four minutes was one of those limitations.

Then Roger Bannister changed history.

Using innovative running strategies that focused on *less* running and more intense, shorter training sessions, in 1954 Bannister did the "impossible" and became the first human being ever to run the mile in less than four minutes. His time: 3:59.4.

But the most amazing things happened *after* Bannister broke the record. Just forty-six days later, his record was broken—and then it was shattered again and again and again. The lesson is an important one, and it has nothing to do with running or the four-minute mile. Bannister had smashed through the real problem that prevents most successes. It's a dark secret that few people ever discuss or admit: most of our barriers are mental. And those mental barriers can place physical and emotional limitations on what you can actually achieve in reality.

Despite the entire world's belief that it wasn't possible to run a mile in less than four minutes, Bannister proved it could be done. His vision and determination opened up the possibilities for everyone to start believing that anything could happen. Once people realized what was possible, it made the rest of the world faster and better.

I want the same to be said about *Evolution*. You'll hear a lot of people say that your body has certain limitations or that your genetics will limit you to looking and feeling a certain way, or that building muscle and shedding fat at the same time is impossible.

Is that what you want for yourself? To believe in a reality where your capabilities are fixed and limited? If that were the case, I would never be where I am today.

My approach is about breaking down perceived limitations by taking a goal, chopping it into smaller pieces in a way that is more easily manageable, and therefore infinitely more doable.

Roger Bannister is an inspiration for all the right reasons. He made the impossible possible by proving that the mind is our worst enemy. In fact, I named my production company "3:59" as a tribute to Bannister's time in the mile and to always remind me of that principle. It is a symbol that anything is possible.

I was always a big kid—and by big, I mean tall. But the truth is, I couldn't have been much weaker when it came to quantifiable strength. In fact, I remember the first time I actually had to "compete" in the weight room during junior high football training. We had a dip bar in a hallway, placed between benches that sat on both sides. Everyone sat on the benches while student after student would walk up to the bar and grind out as many reps as they could.

When it was my turn, I approached the bar assuming I'd place somewhere in the top percentile—only to realize that I didn't have the strength to do a single dip. Think about that the next time you want to assume that I'm built this way due to genetics. I couldn't move my own body weight for one lousy rep, and it pissed me off.

The experience was a harsh wake-up call and the beginning of my own personal battle to rewrite what my body was capable of. I have long limbs, and for lifting weights, that's often considered a curse. I was designed to be lanky, not muscular.

I tried to fight against my body's wishes. I was six foot five in high school but weighed a measly 185 pounds. I desperately wanted to get bigger. I lifted weights. I drank every weight gainer in the world and slugged away day after day, but nothing changed except that I put on a few pounds of fat from all of those extra empty calories.

I continued busting my ass, but nothing seemed to work. I mean, I was always a good athlete. I was the captain of the football, basketball, and volleyball teams from the times I first started playing each. But nonetheless, there I was being singled out by my ninth-grade basketball coaches during my year-end evaluation. I had just led my team in scoring *and* rebounding, but at the bottom of the report was a note: "You need to gain upper-body strength. You need to get stronger."

Where was the praise? The adulation? The gold star? The A-plus? Where was my pat on the back? I'd had a fantastic season, and this was what I got? Criticism? It was embarrassing and frustrating. But they were right. I was left sitting on a bench in the locker room, wondering if it really was impossible for me to gain weight, because it wasn't like I wasn't trying.

Not long afterward, I met my personal Roger Bannister, and everything changed. As you flip through these pages, I realize that you could be the same skinny guy lacking upper-body strength that I was once. But maybe you're not. Maybe you're three hundred pounds and desperate for hope. Or maybe you've been lifting for years, and you've accepted that this is as far as you can go.

It's time to break your four-minute mile.

CHART A NEW COURSE

Around the same time that I was struggling to achieve a single dip or bench-press any type of weight worth bragging about, I noticed a trend in our school. A handful of skinny kids made incredible body transformations after this one particular summer. One of them was my friend and he was huge now, so I asked him what the hell was going on.

It turned out that there was a history teacher at our school named Dr. Jim Mooney, who had trained bodybuilders in the 1970s. He was picking kids who needed a confidence boost, training them in his garage, and transforming them into machines. It was at this point, after endless struggles and the challenge from my coaches, that I made it my mission to find this guy—and convince him to help me out.

I sought out Dr. Mooney, the man who was transforming these kids, and we set up a meeting to speak. My first session was not at all what I expected. It was more like what I imagined a psychological examination for gaining entry into the CIA would be like. His questions were endless. He pulled out medical texts and magazine articles and laid them out, telling me that everything I was doing in the gym, as prescribed by my coaches, was wrong. He came off like a bodybuilding Oliver Stone, weaving his conspiracy theories about the modern state of fitness information. But as I stood there listening for what turned out to be hours, I knew in my gut that this guy was right. He was telling the truth.

I remember vividly Dr. Mooney saying at the end of our session, "If you do this, I need you to be all in. One hundred percent. No questions. I'm not going to waste this knowledge on you if you're the kind of person who dips his toe in, then quits, just so you can turn around and say, 'See, it doesn't work.' You have to trust what I say, and you have to carry it out to the letter." Then in his booming "Moon Dog" voice, he said for the first time what I would come to know as his catchphrase: "I know what I'm doing."

I asked him how he could prove that he could do what seemed impossible. He told me that he would add an inch to my arms in one month. He immediately took out the tape, measured my arm circumference, and we had our baseline.

I told him that I was all in and that I wasn't going to waste his time. I would spend the energy to learn and then apply it.

I jumped up ready to lift, but he told me to come back the next Monday to begin. That week in between the psychological screening and the first workout taught me that training is mental first. You have to get your mind right. You have to get the philosophy right before you jump in.

That following Monday night, we began.

The lifting sessions were unlike anything I'd ever done before. In the beginning, "Moon Dog," as I came to call him, took a page out of Arthur Jones and Dr. Ellington Darden's book. Jones and Darden were two outside-the-box thinkers who created a training philosophy that manifested in the invention and development of the Nautilus machines during the 1970s. Arthur Jones was fascinated by how much strength alligators possessed and from his facility in the Everglades, he recruited Dr. Darden with the hope of creating machines that could train human muscles to function like alligator muscles. Mooney had a full floor of the Nautilus machines in his garage preserved and pristinely maintained, and by using them, he taught me Jones and Darden's philosophy. He had me stop counting reps and sets and start focusing on pushing past physical and mental barriers. For example: I would do chin-ups to failure, and then when I couldn't possibly move my arms, he'd make me do negatives—a physically and mentally challenging process where I would take eight seconds to lower my body on the chin-up bar. It was difficult enough when I was at full strength, but when I was fatigued? It was a special sort of muscle punishment. It literally felt like my biceps were going to rip up through the skin of my arms.

Mooney was resolute in his methodology. His strategy was much like Bannister's: break down the barriers of your mind, and every limitation of your body will cease to exist.

I remember a particular moment when it started to make sense. Moon Dog shared something that Muhammad Ali once said. A reporter came up to Ali after a workout and asked, "How many push-ups can you do?"

Ali, a three-time heavyweight world champion, responded, "About eight or nine."

The reporter looked bewildered. "What? Just eight or nine?"

Ali's answer was along the lines of, "I only start counting when I can't do any more," and then he blasts out another eight or nine.

That's the mentality I had to learn, and it's one of the most important concepts to grasp, in terms of training.

There is fatigue and exhaustion—the point at which most people quit. Those are barriers, not stopping points. You can stop and be good. But what if good is not enough? What if good is really just average? The other option is excellence and superior results. This is the place where few people venture.

Most see a barrier and think that the road is over, instead of realizing that roadblocks in life are really where success begins.

Moon Dog's strategy worked. Sure enough, in a month, my arms were *more* than an inch bigger. And my body kept growing. In fact, my arms grew almost two inches during that initial phase with Mooney. It was a dramatic shift, especially for the other guys on the basketball team. My coaches couldn't believe my transformation, and it was at that time that everyone on the team started calling me "Weider," in reference to the bodybuilding legend Joe Weider.

Hearing that kept me going. It showed me that even though I'd been working hard in all of my workouts previously, my limitations weren't about my genetics; it was about *what* I was doing.

Like Roger Bannister, I saw that something bigger and better was possible for anyone—even a skinny guy like me. The real trick wasn't hidden in reps and sets; it was understanding my body and mind and using that knowledge to learn how to push beyond my comfort level. That's when I started seeing results.

SET THE MIND, AND YOUR BODY WILL FOLLOW

When most people hit the gym, they wonder, "How am I going to make it through this hour?" That's a self-defeating mind-set that would no doubt make any workout difficult—as is approaching your body with the mentality of "How can I ever change?" I want you to forget what you think you know. Throw all that crap in the garbage and develop a case of fitness amnesia.

Approach it like Bannister, who practiced his record-breaking-mile pace in a way that no one had ever tried. He broke the mile into fourths. Once he ran a quarter mile in less than a minute, he then ran two quarter miles in less than a minute each. Eventually, when he could string together four quarters in a row in less than a minute each, he was prepared to show the world and make history.

You can do the same with your body, and that's exactly how we will approach your workouts in *Evolution*. You're going to break down your body into body parts, muscles, sets (the prescribed number of repetitions of an exercise), and reps (short for repetitions, it's the process of performing the exercise. For instance, doing one full chin-up is considered one rep.) And within each rep, you need to put all your energy into the positive motion (lifting the weight) and the negative motion (lowering the weight). Don't worry about anything else. Just focus on the positive and the negative, rep by rep, and keep pushing. When you do that, you will improve.

This is the foundation of *Evolution*. It's an exercise in being present and a lesson that will carry over into every aspect of your life. It's no different than the samurai who practices calligraphy in order to become better at sword fighting. By being in the moment, you teach your mind to stay present, focused, and active, even when you're uncomfortable. You learn to strive for perfection and success at something tiny, such as breathing, pushing, or pulling, yet all of these skills will translate into what you really want: a more impressive, more muscular physique.

The point of this book is to make you better, but before you can move forward, you first need to clear out the clutter. When I was drinking heavily and chain-smoking cigarettes, I was dead in the water. I was never going to know what I could do, because I was chained to an anchor. I couldn't get a fair shot at success unless I could somehow find a way to saw through that chain. I had to learn how to get out of my own way in order to fully realize my potential.

For years when I was young, people said, "You have so much potential." I used to be flattered by it. But, as I got older, I realized that *potential* is a negative word. It meant that there was something—or a lot—that I hadn't reached. For a while, I tried to see what I could get away with, and it wasn't until later that there was a paradigm shift into *"What can I actually do? What can I actually achieve?"*

I'm not eighteen anymore, but you will never hear me whine about it. I'm thirty-six now, almost thirty-seven, and I'm in better shape than I've ever been in my life—physically and mentally. You might think that you're too skinny to pack on size. Or you might believe you're too fat to push your body. Maybe you're intimidated by the gym. Whatever is holding you back, we're going to figure it out—together—so you can inhabit the body and life that you want. It is achievable. It is possible.

You can start your entire life over today.

I want you to understand something very important: no one walks into the gym ripped on day one. Even Arnold was a skinny fifteen-year-old in Thal, Austria, trying to find his way around a weight rack. The gym is the great equalizer. Everyone there deserves respect, no matter what his or her shape, size, or level of development. To me, everyone is on the same ground, working hard to become better. The fact that you showed up is all that anyone worth a damn cares about, and it's all you need to instantly earn respect for yourself and respect from me.

One time at a gym in Arizona, I was working out when I spotted this little kid. He was on the preacher bench—the slanted bench that supports your arms so they hang at a 45-degree angle to your body—doing curls with perfect form and a professional level of focus. After each set, he would put down the bar, and pick up a little notebook and pen he kept next to him, and log everything in detail.

I stood there for a minute watching him go through his routine. He was busting his ass like a grown man, even though he was a boy. I laughed to myself at how rad this kid was. I had so much respect for what he was doing. He was unknowingly putting to shame most of the adults who were dicking around on their cell phones, having conversations while sitting on pieces of equipment. If I could buy "life stock" in this kid, I would, because given the way he went about his workout, I guarantee that if you check back in on him ten or twenty years down the line, he's going to be running shit.

The lesson here: In order for you to become "the Man," you first have to be *that kid*. He's hustling, he's got his workout gear on, and he doesn't give a shit what I'm lifting or how much weight I'm putting up. He's too busy, head down, focusing on himself and following his plan.

If he follows it long enough and takes all the steps, that kid is going to get what he deserves.

You've got to enter the gym devoid of shame and comparison. You're entering into a competition of one: yourself. Once you walk through those doors, no one is going to make fun of you for not lifting enough or doing something wrong. The gym is a community of people working together to become better, instead of accepting their fate as predetermined: "I'm built this way or that way, and nothing I do is going to change that."

My trainer since 2010, Ron Mathews, was also the kid, like me, who couldn't do one pull-up or dip in high school. Ron is in his midforties now, and he is an absolute beast. Up until two years ago, he was still playing tight end for the number two–ranked semipro football team in America. This year, he competed in the CrossFit Games—a competition that tests strength, speed, and endurance of some of the best athletes in the world—and placed ninth in the world for men over forty! Instead of looking at the people who are where you want to be and accepting that it's not part of your fate, you need to take a hard look and see where you can go next.

A few years ago, I was moving and clearing out some boxes when I found an old *Men's Health* magazine I'd bought in 2003. I remember seeing it on the rack and thinking, "I want to be built like that guy on the cover." So I bought it, and somehow, over the years, it had found its way into that box. I couldn't believe my eyes when I realized that the guy on the cover was none other than my trainer, Ron. Here it was seven years later, and I was being trained by the exact guy who represented my fitness goals. Coincidence? I don't think so.

In order to find your path, sometimes it's not always the positive examples that can push you down the road. Sometimes it's incredibly motivating to look at who or what frustrates you and get angry about it. I've always been a huge proponent of using resentment as rocket fuel. I've learned in life that my jealousy and envy can provide a useful compass pointing me toward my goals.

I remember being in high school, sitting on the couch with my girlfriend watching MTV, and the video for "Under the Bridge" by the Red Hot Chili Peppers came on. The video ends with a shirtless Anthony Kiedis running in slow motion, long hair swinging, pecs bouncing, and the room got silent—*loud* silent. I looked over at my girlfriend and realized that she was practically drooling over this guy. Here I was, a fifteen-year-old with short, preppy hair and a sunken chest that wouldn't grow. I felt the anger come over me. I *hated* this guy, and for years I couldn't stand the Chilis. Anytime anyone brought them up, I got angry. What was causing my jealousy? Simple: my unmet potential.

As an adult, I can look back and laugh. I *love* the Red Hot Chili Peppers. They are one of my all-time favorite bands! I've seen them in concert a bunch of times, and I've even met Kiedis on more than one occasion. I can say that he is one of the coolest dudes I've ever met. That guy busted his ass for everything he has, and he deserves all of his success. I was just a kid who needed to stop whining and being a hater and get up off of that couch and start working up to my potential. It took me a while, but I eventually found the way to turn it all into positive energy.

The funny thing is that twenty-plus years later, I'm guessing there is some guy somewhere sitting on a couch looking at me with my long hair, running around shirtless in the woods on *True Blood* or in my fireman costume in *Magic Mike,* absolutely hating my guts.

It's those resentments and insecurities that oftentimes can steer you exactly where you need to go.

CHAPTER 3

Taking
Action

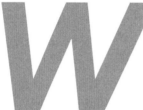

When I take on a new part, I approach it with meticulous attention to detail. Take my role as Alcide Herveaux on *True Blood*. As soon as I was cast, I broke down the character into pieces. First there was the geographic layer. On the show, Alcide is from Jackson, Mississippi, which meant that I was going to be speaking in a Jackson dialect, as well as portraying a set of southern values that are slightly different from those elsewhere. I enlisted the help of one of the best dialect coaches on the planet, who also happened to be the head of the voice and speech program at the Carnegie Mellon School of Drama, prior to my attending there. We pored over CD after CD of people from Mississippi, until I found a model that sounded right for Alcide. We then used the phonetic alphabet that I was drilled to death on in drama school to break every line of dialogue into syllabic pieces consisting of vowel and consonant sounds, so that I could start to learn the unique speech patterns native to the region.

Next came the spiritual and mental sides to him. I used *The Southern Vampire Mysteries* by Charlaine Harris—the novels that *True Blood* is based on—to create a backstory for his past, to connect the dots of why he thinks and feels the way he does.

After the internal work, I then turned to developing the physical. Alcide is a man who shares DNA with wolves, so I watched and read everything I could get my hands on pertaining to wolves. I even found a way to spend time with and observe real wolves. On top of that, I got a tan, because my character is used to working and being outside, and also to further separate my character from the cold, corpse-like vampires he would be up against.

Last but not least, I wanted my body to look ripped and sinewy, like an animal's. I knew that the more physically imposing I was, the more that would offset how sensitive and romantic he is. I wanted to look stronger than an average human, which called for stronger-than-average effort. So I enlisted Ron Mathews, who is the same man who got Hugh Jackman in shape for *X-Men*, and the rest is history.

While the task might seem bizarre—or completely inapplicable to you—the way I handled the situation is an important lesson in turning a goal into an action and, inevitably, into a success.

My transformation into a werewolf was calculated. I tried to figure out the components of what was needed to play the role of a half-man, half-beast construction contractor from Jackson, Mississippi, who hates what he is.

While you might not be training to become a werewolf, the point I'm making has to do with approach. It's the same success formula I've used to transform my body and make improvements year after year.

The more specific you are about planning and goals, the better your results will be. For the movie *Sabotage* with Arnold, I prepared for my role of Joseph "Grinder" Phillips, a U.S. Drug Enforcement Administration agent who works undercover in a biker gang. I read a book about a former college football player turned ATF (Bureau of Alcohol, Tobacco, and Firearms) agent who'd posed as a biker and infiltrated the Hells Angels in real life. I looked at photos of him and used them as the inspiration for what I wanted my character to look like physically. He looked like a linebacker. He was a thick-necked former college football player now covered in tattoos: big and scary. So I told Ron my goal, and we adjusted my training to achieve it. I did more Olympic lifting, such as dead lifts, cleans, and presses, and stole tricks from powerlifting. As a result, I put on twenty pounds in about two months and was the biggest I had ever been.

When I was preparing to play the male stripper "Big Dick Richie" in *Magic Mike*, the goal was simple: be straight-up ripped and shredded. The plan, therefore, focused on a lot of conditioning and eliminating the rest periods during my workouts. I also had to plan for filming shirtless every day for weeks at a time, which provided a huge challenge that we will get into in greater detail in chapter 9, when I talk about shoots and filming.

I recommend that you prepare the same way. List your goals. Determine your next steps and then break *those* next steps into next steps. This book includes a starter program—the exact same one that prepared me for my first season on *True Blood*. Whether you want to become bigger and stronger or more cut up and shredded, I've done the work for you. But *you* are the only one in control of your focus. Remember, it's the mental blocks that hold most people back. Goal setting is one of the biggest mental aspects of training, and yet it often gets overlooked. So, with the help of my trainer, Ron, we put together the most efficient plan possible. It's a step-by-step guide that will allow you to set your goals, get out of your own way, and step into the body and life you've always wanted.

THE RULES OF GOAL SETTING

I have always struggled with pull-ups. My long arms have made them the bane of my existence. I know this, so here's what I *don't* do on day one in the gym: say I'm going to do thirty pull-ups and just magically expect to do them, and then, when I don't achieve that goal, assume that I'm a failure. Thirty pull-ups is my *end* goal, not my *first* goal. Part of being successful is creating "first goals." It's the old "You have to crawl before you can walk" mentality. But what I want is for you to get to the walk phase faster than you ever thought possible.

In terms of the thirty pull-ups, I'd set up a plan to help you reach one. Or five. Or ten. No matter the goal, there is always a path. You just have to choose to walk down it.

Not being able to do a single dip or pull-up could be the best thing that ever happened to you. It means you'll have to devise a program to do just one by making every muscle in your body that much stronger. Then you'll move on to two, and three, and four. It's harder to first get your body into motion than it is to keep up the momentum.

You are going to have to let it hurt. Let it suck. Arnold purposefully wouldn't cover body parts he hated, in order to motivate himself. Don't deny your weaknesses. Use them as fuel.

You need to create goals that will make you uncomfortable. Most people are not okay with that. I like to say that in order to be successful, you need to "let the baby cry in the crib." What I mean by that is that we all have this part of us that wants to cry out and complain when things get tough or quit when something feels uncomfortable. But in reality, if there's nothing to cry about—if the baby's diaper is clean, and it's been fed—that little voice needs to learn to be quiet. This may take practice, but it's never tougher than the first time around.

The moment you can embrace that discomfort is the moment when you'll start really succeeding at those smaller goals and setting yourself up on the path to bigger things.

When I was cast on *True Blood*, I wasn't thinking about being on the list of *Men's Health* 100 Best Physiques of All Time, alongside my childhood heroes Bo Jackson and Michael Jordan. It wasn't about starring in a movie with Arnold or getting a fitness-book deal. It started with wanting to get into the best shape I'd ever been in and then trying to improve on that step by step. I put all of my energy into the footwork, and the path revealed itself. I kept busy setting smaller goal after smaller goal on my way to something bigger. I constantly pushed back the finish line, in order to stay hungry and see just how much I could achieve if I kept on pushing.

I challenge you to create that mind-set for yourself. Many people set goals, but very few really give themselves the chance to find out what they are truly capable of. The exhilaration of pushing limits, rather than setting ceilings, can lead to some amazing things that can surprise even the biggest of dreamers.

AVOIDING THE TRAPS AND FINDING YOUR EDGE

In the book *The War of Art: Break Through the Blocks and Win Your Inner Creative Battles*, Steven Pressfield identifies all the different types of resistance that people face. The most important takeaway: the amateur quits, while the professional fights through.

The same applies to mastering your body and getting into the best shape of your life.

Sometimes people look at me like I'm an alien for training the way that I do, and the questions I get make me laugh:

"Why can't you just eat that?"

"Does that really make that much of a difference?"

"Why do you still train so hard?"

"You can skip a day, right?"

"Can I substitute exercises in the program?"

Dealing with people's insecurities about their own health and fitness can be the most difficult aspect of training. Sometimes, unfortunately, that can come in the form of family, friends, and loved ones. Which is why you need people around you who are supportive of you getting fit. I've had ex-girlfriends who were so bogged down with their own baggage that they could not for the life of them get on board with what I was trying to accomplish. They were threatened by my commitment to training and diet. Apparently my getting fitter was shining a spotlight on their shortcomings. How did I know this? Because they told me so—sometimes very loudly and sometimes in extremely subtle fashion. Rather than choose to be inspired by me, those people made my already difficult mission even tougher. You're either in the boat, or you're not.

During my first season on *True Blood*, I had the privilege of working with all-around great guy Don Swayze. During a rehearsal of one of our werewolf fight scenes, Don shared with me that a few years prior he'd had a crazy accident base jumping at night and shattered his leg in seventy-two places. As a result of the accident, the bones in his leg were replaced with steel rods, a steel plate was placed in his pelvis, and the front part of his foot was removed. He had been an avid skydiver his whole life, and that love eventually led him to the dangerous sport of base jumping. I shared with Don that I had been skydiving two days in a row with the army's parachute team, the Golden Knights, and absolutely loved it! In fact, the guys on the team offered to tutor me through the skydiving certification process, but my girlfriend at the time was horrified at the thought of me ever doing it again. To this Don replied, "There're plenty of other women out there who love skydiving, my man." Don loved skydiving, and he could have easily let it be taken from him and settled for a life devoid of what he loved the most. Everyone in their right mind would have understood, but that's not what he did. Don continued jumping through it all and managed to log one thousand skydiving jumps with a cast on his foot! I bet that as I write this, after thirteen surgeries and twenty-two months on crutches, Don Swayze is out there somewhere right now either jumping or planning his next jump.

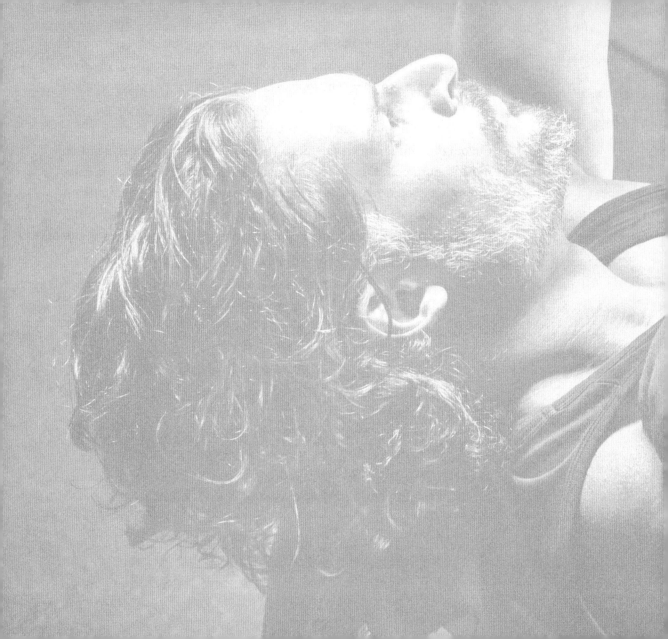

CHAPTER 4

The New Rules of Exercise

have the privilege of spending a lot of time on the road. And by that, I mean that I'm able to see the world, meet lots of different people, and observe different cultures and habits, both in the United States and abroad. Throughout all of those travels and places I've visited, I've noticed a common denominator in terms of fitness: people have no idea what they are doing in the gym.

It's not just a lack of effort that's the problem. It's a lack of knowledge—in terms of what exercises to do, how to do them, and how hard you need to push to see the type of results you hope to achieve.

People want things easy. They want a magic pill. My greatest example of this is the escalator. An invention of the twentieth century, it's basically an electric staircase that moves roughly as fast as—that's right, a person walking up a flight of stairs. So what do people do? Stand on it, enabling them to get to their destination at the same time they would have without it, minus the exercise. That's the world we live in.

Maybe it has always been that way, and I'm just late to the party.

The famous psychologist Carl Jung wrote essays about his fear that technology was increasing at such a rapid rate that if morality didn't increase at an equal rate, we would eventually end up in a very difficult position. That is exactly what I see happening, especially when it comes to fitness and today's work ethic.

Standing on the shoulders of Jung is the legendary Joe Weider.

JOE WEIDER: VISIONARY

Joe Weider was a futuristic thinker and doer. It was in the July 1950 issue of *Your Physique* that he made these ten predictions concerning bodybuilding's impact on the future of health. It's amazing how right he got it, even way back then.

1. "I predict that civilization will speed up in every phase, and that the stresses and strains on mankind will continue to increase."

2. "I predict that the resulting increase in mental and physical illness will force the world to recognize the importance of systematic exercise and physical activities."

3. "I predict that bodybuilding will become the chief form of systematic exercise and physical activity, and that it will come to be looked upon as one of the greatest forces in the field of preventive medicine."

4. "I predict that a full realization of the importance of muscular development will sweep the world, and the sport of bodybuilding will grow by leaps and bounds."

5. "I predict that the principles of good bodybuilding—which include a balanced diet, adequate sleep, plenty of fresh air, ample sunshine, and regular workouts—will become basic principles of living."

6. "I predict that bodybuilding will become the stepping-stone to every other sport and physical activity."

7. "I predict that the art of relaxation, one of the fundamental principles in bodybuilding, will become more and more important as tensions increase, and that relaxation will be universally taught and advocated."

8. "I predict that bodybuilding will spread to every corner of the world and that it will one day be recognized as the king of all sports and physical activities."

9. "I predict that those who practice bodybuilding will live healthier, happier, and more useful lives."

10. "I predict that bodybuilding will one day become one of the greatest forces in existence, and that it may be hailed as the activity that actually saved civilization from itself."

The technologies that we have created are doing our bodies a disservice. A great example is how many gyms have many circuit machines but no Olympic weight platforms and rubber plates. This is not a complete admonishment of machines, but this approach caters only to people who don't know what they're doing. Relying on machines propagates a myth of "Do a few of these, a few of these, and you're done." The industry is based on making you think that newer is better. It's about selling equipment rather than getting results for the people using them. I do want to be clear: those machines are infinitely better than sitting on the couch. But this book provides what you really need: a program to maximize your gains for the amount of effort you expend.

TAKING BACK THE GYM AND ENDING ALL THAT IS WRONG

This book is about looking and feeling better, but that doesn't mean it's purely about aesthetics. Yes, I can teach you to burn fat and build muscle. But training the right way goes beyond that. It will make you a better person; you'll be healthier, move better, and become a better athlete. You'll build self-esteem and confidence. Studies have shown that rigorous exercise is just as effective as the drug Prozac in battling depression. You will also benefit from increased energy and vitality.

Training the right way is the fountain of youth.

Too many people emphasize the bathroom scale and mirror. If you want to hit the right number on the scale and see the best possible image in the mirror, you need to shift your focus *away* from those elements. Instead, focus on progress, selecting the right exercises, moving better, lifting more, working harder, and then repeating all of those processes. When you do that, everything will change, and the scale and mirror will follow.

In order to make permanent changes, you need to instill habits that will allow you to replicate your efforts. You want to feel good and be motivated by your program, but what you may not understand is that it's *not* going to feel good, especially at the beginning. You're not automatically going to want to take these steps and do this program, because it's going to be harder than what you've been told works.

If you stick with it through the pain and discomfort, and do it repeatedly, your body will get to a point of wanting it. Your reward will be a desire to do it after all the times of not wanting to do it, but you won't get to that reward phase until you push through the tough stuff.

It will happen for you. You just have to change your mind-set and push through. I didn't get a book deal and *then* start working out—or swear to put in twenty-five years of working out in return.

The beautiful thing about fitness is that nowhere else are you going to find an activity that is so responsive to your effort. Everything having to do with your body, you have to earn. The results are completely up to you and are quantifiable almost immediately. I see people shortchange themselves constantly, saying, "This isn't me." But it absolutely could be.

That's why I'm excited to give this program to the public. I believe it can change anybody. Work this program solid for eight to twelve weeks, like I did preparing for the first season of *True Blood*, and you can turn into an animal too.

I'm lucky in that I've had mentors and trainers who told it to me like it is. I know I speak for them when I say that the best information shouldn't be limited to the lucky few. It shouldn't be saved for athletes and celebrities. The ability to build muscle and burn fat is not a privilege, so why hide the "secrets"? These benefits are earned, so you should be armed with the right information that will give you the chance to earn them.

I'm an actor. I'm not here to sell fitness products or gimmicky workouts. I'm a guy who has never touched an anabolic steroid or human growth hormone, who has trained with some of the best trainers on the planet, and who wants to deliver to you what I *know* works, without any useless crap.

I've stolen fire from the gods and I'm giving it to you. What you do with it is up to you.

The last thing I want to do is rush you and throw you into a workout expecting instant success. That's the mistake that nearly every fitness book makes. If it were as simple as *just* giving you a list of exercises, a lot more people would be in shape.

My trainer, Ron, and I agree that the hardest thing for most people to wrap their brains around is the fact that they don't have an accurate frame of reference for what intensity is. *Real* intensity. Everything is based on their own experience, which makes complete sense, but if your own perception of "hard" is what you set as your threshold, you may never really understand just how much you can achieve. This goes back to Roger Bannister. We all have that four-minute-mile perception in some way with our bodies. But you know what? No one has ever hit a workout harder than they ever did before and then not been able to get back to that level again. Sure, you might need more rest or recovery, but you need to learn to start going beyond what you think is your maximum effort. In order to move forward, you need to fathom how hard a workout can be. I'm guessing that right now you walk out of the gym feeling good and invigorated, yet your results are middle of the road. I'm suggesting that the results you really want lie somewhere in the ballpark of crawling or staggering out to your car with your arms shaking so badly, you're barely able to pull your car keys out of your pocket and hold the steering wheel steady on the drive home.

Truth: You think you're working out at an 8. You're actually at a 2. I don't care how long you've been training; that's just the reality. If that hurts your feelings, I'm sorry. It's time for you to reestablish your baseline in order to define intensity.

In exercise science, intensity is equal to your power. The equation for power is simple:

$$[\text{Force} \times \text{distance}] / \text{time} = \text{power}$$

You don't need to be a biophysicist to see how this translates to fitness. Learning how to increase your power means manipulating one of three variables: more weight, less rest in between exercises, or more reps. All of these adjustments will make you improve.

In other words, it's time to focus on exertion. If you're always exerting more power, you'll keep getting better session after session. And that's when you see changes.

In order to get to that point, you need to reset your perception and your approach to the "rules" that will in turn make you look better. I can tell you right now, it's not what you think it is.

WHAT REALLY WORKS

Walk into any gym, and it becomes apparent very quickly how most guys approach their workouts. Guys like lifting heavy weights. It's what they do. But how they go about it is completely wrong. You see too many men working their way up to one heavy set and then resting for four minutes between sets. That's too much rest. Or maybe they'll repeat that heavy weight for a few sets, take it to failure, and then move on to the next exercise.

Sure, you might get stronger, but how do you look in the mirror? Are you really any closer to your goals?

I know you're not, because I was once in your shoes. One of the biggest eye-openers for me occurred when I started working with Ron. I was in this place where I would always default to heavy weights. When I met Ron that first day, I weighed in at 240 pounds, but on camera I looked doughy. I'm sure I could lift more than just about any actor you could find, but the camera didn't care about that. Cameras pick up the separation and shadows between muscles, so our goal right away was to cut it all down so that my muscles would look more defined on the screen. The lighter the weights and more cardio I did, the better I would end up looking.

I wanted to look the biggest and most beastly I'd ever looked. Ron's response? "Cardio, cardio, cardio, intensity, intensity, intensity." Exactly what I didn't want to hear. I was afraid that I would flatten out my size by slogging away on a treadmill for hours on end.

I couldn't have been more wrong.

Ron's program cut twenty pounds off of me in eight weeks, while increasing every single muscle measurement on my body and reducing my waist size. That first year on *True Blood*, I had to have all of my suit jackets tailored *twice*, due to the amount my muscles were growing.

This new way to train is about pushing intensity. If you want to gain size *and* burn fat without being a slave to cardio, you need to work harder, faster, and more efficiently. The workouts you'll find in chapter 6 will give you a cardio workout while you lift weights. You'll raise your heart rate and find new ways to become stronger. It's a concept known as metabolic resistance training, and CrossFit has recently popularized the method. Do big-muscle exercises at a rapid pace while trying to maintain the highest intensity possible for as long as possible. Once the intensity drops below a certain level, you stop.

Yes: you keep fighting once you get tired, but eventually you get to the point where you need to shut it down, because the intensity will be too low to see results. Then the next time, you bring even more to your workout. Rinse and repeat. Eventually the bar of intensity—of weight, of distance, and of shorter rest periods—all improve. Combine that with some strategic cardio, and you will be ripped in no time.

WHY IT WORKS

This might seem to go against the conventional wisdom of "Go hard or go home," but going hard doesn't just mean that you lift as much weight as humanly possible. Yes, you want to get strong, but in a strategic manner. Consider this sample workout: we set a timer for ten minutes and start by doing three reps of clean and press—an exercise where you pull a barbell from shin height up to your shoulders and then press the weight overhead—followed by three reps of pull-ups. Then you do six reps of each. Followed by nine and then twelve.

Now, the odds are that you won't work your way all the way up to twelve reps of each exercise, but for the sake of this experiment, just consider what's happening within these ten minutes. On the clean and press, you're working every muscle in your body. You're pulling a weight in a vertical pattern and then dropping down to a squat to work your lower body. Then you stand up and press the weight overhead.

After those weights, you move to pull-ups, one of the best upper-body pulling exercises. It's working your back, your arms, your chest, and your core—which includes your abs and lower back.

In terms of exercise movements (that is, the directions in which you can move weights), you cover four of the biggest patterns: (1) vertical pull for your upper and lower body (the first part of the clean), (2) vertical push for your legs (the squatting), (3) vertical push for your upper body (the overhead press), and (4) vertical pull (the pull-ups).

MOVEMENT PATTERNS

Vertical push	**Overhead press, push press, military press, squat**
Vertical pull	**Chin-up, pull-up, lat pull-down**
Horizontal push	**Bench press, incline press**
Horizontal pull	**Bent-over row, seat cable row, dumbbell row**
Rotational	**Core twist**

Not only do you move in many of the major movement patterns, you also hit all of the major muscle groups. On the first part of the clean, you work the back of your legs (hamstrings, gluteus muscles, or glutes), and your upper back, including your trapezius muscles (traps). On the second part of the clean, you challenge the front side of your legs (quadriceps, or quads). The press then takes care of your shoulders (all three deltoid muscles), and the pull-ups finish off the rest of your body.

So while the "workout" might last only ten minutes, you start seeing how quickly you can push your entire body in ways that used to take hours.

This was the biggest eye-opener: how much work we'd get done in a short period of time. Because remember, the goal is to not stop. We want to minimize the time element of the power equation. So rather than predetermined long periods of rest, sometimes you'll be resting only as needed—or not resting at all. And we'll organize workouts in a way so that we don't have to stop unnecessarily.

This method challenges your cardio in a way that burns fat, pushes your muscles so that you can gain size, and allows you only enough strategic rest to keep up intensity.

CHECK YOUR EGO

If you're anything like me, something might occur to you while digesting this new approach: "How the hell am I supposed to lift these heavy weights without rest?"

Simple: you don't. At least, not at first. You drop the weight. You drop your ego, and you watch your body transform.

When I first shifted to this new model of training, I struggled from the mental standpoint. I wanted to be the big, strong guy in the gym at all times. But no matter how heavy I lifted, the moment I took off my shirt, the results were not what I wanted.

I was still stuck in this mind-set that the only quantifiable measurement for progress was weight. I couldn't hear anything else. Yet by breaking down my mechanics and focusing on higher intensity through less rest, I was forced to go back to square one. By doing so, I was able to catch up to speed pretty quickly and rocket forward to lift more than ever before. I had to undo my weak foundation, because the skyscraper I had dreamed of building on it was turning out to be more of a town house.

If you'd like some help shifting your mind-set, here's a tip from Arnold: resistance is resistance is resistance. Your muscles don't know if the weight is heavy or not. Your muscles go on and go off. You use only as many fibers as your muscles need. So working at a moderate weight and learning how to completely turn on that muscle fiber is more beneficial than just stacking a bar with weight and putting tension on your ligaments and joints to control the movement. The goal is to squeeze your muscles during each movement, and for every rep to be controlled and felt in your muscles through a full range of motion. And for that to happen, you need to drop the weight. Check your ego, lower the weight, and let your body grow.

Then when you can go heavier with the weights, you're going to receive the full benefits. For instance, on an exercise like the bench press, you're pushing primarily from your chest, not from your shoulders or arms or latissimus dorsi muscles (lats). By cheating, you can think you're succeeding, because you're lifting more. But in actuality, you're not using the muscles that are intended, and as a result, you're not making the body part work as hard as it can. Create the mind–muscle connection first and *then* increase the weight.

This paradigm shift may be an uncomfortable one, but trust me: the sooner you can let go of looking around the gym and thinking, "Why is that guy lifting that much more weight than me?" the better off you'll be. The only person you are now in competition with is *you*. The harder you work, the better you will look. Your appearance isn't parallel to how heavy you lift, it's parallel to how hard you work. If you keep pushing the intensity, in time you'll look great *and* be stronger.

I don't believe in taking every set to failure. That is, you shouldn't take every set to the point where you absolutely, positively can't move your muscles at all. There is a time and place for failure training, but not in every set of every workout.

This comes with a big caveat: most people don't know the point of failure. They shut themselves down prematurely and assume they can't do more. The more that you can push your body when it's fatigued—while maintaining good form and keeping the tension in your muscles—the better. Those are the reps that are going to help you look the way you want to look.

These are what I call the "money reps." Money reps are where you earn your paycheck. They're the reps late in a set or a workout when your muscles are burning and fatigued and screaming at you to quit. I'm here to let you know that they're not signaling you to stop; they're calling you out, to push yourself harder, to break through your barriers, to turn off the pain, and to grow and transform your body. Instead of thinking, "Oh God, this is going to hurt," you should be thinking, "I've got my body on the run. This is the point where I chase it down and force my muscles to grow."

A lot of people train and have no idea what failure is. They don't know what training at that top 10 percent effort feels like. So push your boundaries! Not to actual failure, mind you, but to *technical* failure. Find that place where you actually run out of gas and your form breaks down. Then get some well-earned rest, so that you can bounce back harder the next time.

NEXT-LEVEL FITNESS

I realize that a lot of people might not even know what pushing past fatigue feels like. So Ron Mathews and I designed a test that will teach you intensity and mental strength, so that you can begin to practice breaking down your mental boundaries.

Try any one of these physical tests, each one increasing in difficulty. Remember, the goal is to not quit.

TEST 1: FORTY PUSH-UPS WITHOUT STOPPING
Tip: When you tire, you can hold yourself in the plank position. This will challenge your core while giving you a small break.

TEST 2: ONE HUNDRED BODY-WEIGHT SQUATS WITHOUT RESTING

TEST 3: THIRTY PULL-UPS WITHOUT LETTING GO OF THE BAR
Tip: You might want to use chalk or tape your hands. This is tough.

Remember, it's not what you can do in one workout. Or even what you can do in four weeks or three months. It's bigger than that. So learn to push your limits now, and every workout for the rest of your life will be exponentially better. Every set and rep will carry more weight. Your best body will have no choice but to follow.

Intensity alone is not enough. You can have a great workout where you push the limits of the power equation and still not end up where you want. That's because two more key elements are mind-set and focus. Intensity is dependent on your ability to zone in and push yourself without any other distractions. When you're at work, if you multitask too much, your production suffers. In your personal life, if you're oblivious and distracted, your relationships suffer. If you're in the gym and your mind is on something else while you're working out, your results suffer. That is what undercuts most training sessions.

Focus is the most important variable because it determines your ability to give everything to your workout. It allows you to make sure that you don't get hurt and that you're able to keep pushing your limits. Once you do go high weight, fear is going to rear its head. I get nervous when I go heavy sometimes, especially with squats and dead lifts. But over time, I've learned to gauge my fatigue level. When I get exhausted, it becomes a mental struggle to keep good form, and therefore, I run a higher risk of suffering a pinched nerve or a muscle tear. Good focus is so important because it allows you to insure good form and go up in weight without causing injury.

I remember when I suffered one of my more frustrating injuries. I pinched a nerve between the fifth and sixth cervical vertebrae in my neck because I got tired, sloppy, and wasn't concentrating. Focus takes on greater importance as you break in to this new style of workout. The tendency is to concentrate less as sets and reps go on, which is exactly when you most need to lock in your mind on the exercise. Fight to maintain your posture and form at all times.

Think about it this way: you're operating heavy machinery. Focus!

Lifting weights is incredibly mental. It entails focusing on your body parts and then honing in on the specific muscles. It involves breathing and staying calm, while applying your concentrated energy to the iron. There is a Zen-like quality to training, but it can be appreciated only when you put yourself in the right mind-set.

THE PSYCHOLOGY OF BODY TRANSFORMATION

It's important to come clean and accept the fears and doubts that you admit only to yourself. Identify the blocks in your life. I find that most people "try not to fail." They never reach success because they fear the sacrifices it might take to get there. It looks crazy when you see it written out like that, but self-sabotage is public enemy number one if you ask me, as well as a modern plague of the spirit.

Most people are satisfied with "pretty good." When they reach it, they become complacent, and they never become hungry for that next level. While you're training on this program, I want to remind you not to stop at average. You have to tell yourself that you can do it ten times better than you've ever done before. Self-sabotage is a form of fear, and, like water, it takes the form of whatever it encounters. Depending on where you are in a given situation, that will determine the form you will face:

You're too tired.

You're too sore.

You don't feel like warming up.

You don't feel like pushing through extra reps.

You cut the workout short.

You find yourself making excuses.

You allow peers to influence and undermine your goals.

You begin to doubt that it will work.

You stop caring about your program and making progress on your body.

These barriers are real, but don't let them become excuses. If you were an actor, and Steven Soderbergh called and said he wanted you for his next movie, but, "Oh, by the way, you're playing a male stripper named 'Big Dick Richie' and you're going to be almost naked the entire time," what would you do? You'd get your ass in shape!

You might not be an actor, but that's the example I want you to imagine and aspire to. In order to achieve a certain level of success, first find a certain level of motivation.

It's the one thing I can't give you in this book. I can teach you everything else, but I can't teach that desire. Whatever your fears or blocks are, you need to find a motivation bigger than them. I can't determine the thing most important to you that will keep that fire burning when you have those moments of doubt. Once you have that, I can help you. If you don't have it, I can only match what you bring. Commitment = desire + action. The bigger the desire, the better the results.

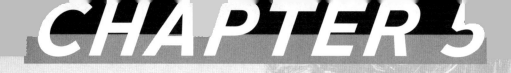

CHAPTER 5

Preparing
for **Your**
New
Body

When Arnold Schwarzenegger wrote *The New Encyclopedia of Modern Bodybuilding*, he created a comprehensive blueprint to guide men toward a better body. It broke down everything we knew at the time about working your muscles and making them grow.

When we try to figure out what real advances we've made since then, what's most frustrating is sifting through the mountains of misinformation. When you really get into it, we've moved away from a lot of the techniques that worked just fine. That's why when it comes to modern fitness, in many ways we've got to go backward to progress.

We need a new approach that takes a look back at the things that worked while putting a new spin on them, using the advances that have been made in the past twenty years. Combining an old-school philosophy with some new-school knowledge.

The Russians in the 1950s and the bodybuilders of the 1960s and '70s pretty much had it figured out. But rather than evolve the best ideas into something better, experts look for something new (and usually inferior) because they need to make money. It's a flawed dynamic that has led us down a road of gimmicks, misinformation, and lots of frustration. The perfect example is all of the late-night infomercials for fitness devices being peddled by some celebrity and being demonstrated by a bunch of fitness models whose physiques were obviously not molded and shaped by the brand-new products they're selling. We live in a capitalist society. I get it, but my primary goal in writing this book is not to make money (I make plenty at my day job). It's about setting the record straight and giving the public the truth.

My approach starts with making a list of everything that works, and then showing you ways to improve on them—but, in some cases, not adjusting a thing. If it ain't broke, don't fix it. This book is a compilation of what I've gathered from the best fitness minds on the planet, and my physique was created by using nothing other than what you see here.

THE TIMELINE

Every person is motivated in a different way. Some people respond to positive feedback and others to negative. Having a coach or trainer yell and scream might amp you up and push you to another level, while for others, it would crush them and leave them crippled and unable to move forward.

No matter who you are and what you respond to, you can push forward as long as you are realistic and adjust for your experience level. It requires an honest inventory and assessment of "Where am I right now?"

Are you a beginner? If so, you probably haven't been training at all recently, or you have less than two years of experience. Less than two years of pumping iron, in my mind, still makes you a beginner. So check your ego, don't take it personally, and realize that a hungry and humble attitude will serve you more in the end.

Are you intermediate? If so, you've been hitting the gym *consistently* for three to six years. You know how to push yourself and stay *consistent*. Fitness is already a lifestyle for you and you're looking to take it up a notch or two.

Are you advanced? At this point, you've been in the iron game for more than seven years. You work hard, you push the limits, but you want more because you know there's more to be had. You understand that you're still just scratching the surface, and you want to know exactly what you can become.

Remember, realistic expectations lead to realistic goals, which create real results.

For instance, in Olympic sprinting, everything is separated by hundredths of a second. It's such a small amount, but making up that tiny gap requires a world of effort. The lesson being: whenever you get closer to the top and inch closer to your ultimate goals, the harder it will be to progress. Remember that, and you'll have fewer doubts when the changes don't come as quickly anymore. That mind-set alone will put you ahead of 99 percent of the people out there trying to change how they look. The closer you get to the top of Mount Everest, the harder it is to breathe in that altitude. It's always the last few steps to the summit that can feel like an eternity. Likewise, the closer you get to physical perfection, the harder the training sessions get.

FIND YOUR PATH: WHAT TO EXPECT IN THE WORKOUTS

PHASE 1: INCORPORATE (WEEKS 1–2)

When it comes to training, everything starts and ends with understanding your muscles and which ones you want to use to move the weight. Many people think that gyms are filled with mirrors for reasons of vanity—and judging by the alarming number of douche-y guys at the gym lifting their shirts in the "Situation" pose, flexing their abs, I can see why. The actual functional purpose of the mirrors is to help you focus on the muscles you're working. They are there to facilitate the mind–muscle connection. On each curl, your job is to squeeze and activate every last fiber of your biceps. On the bench press, you want to hone in on the range of motion so that you stretch the muscle at the bottom and squeeze your pecs at the top, keeping tension on your muscles and not your joints. It's much easier to fire off each muscle and focus on the contraction when you can see it.

Squeezing and contracting muscles might seem like common sense when you see it in writing, but it's actually one of the most commonly overlooked aspects of training—even by those who would consider themselves advanced. This is what bodybuilders understand from posing: how to squeeze every muscle and activate it. It's important, because it teaches you how to listen to your body. At the beginner level, your primary directive is to increase your mind–muscle connection and learn to squeeze and activate every single muscle group at will.

In order to learn, it will take practice and patience. They say it takes a broken bone eight weeks to hard wire fully so that you can exert yourself confidently once again. It will take about that long to adapt to how to really train.

When you start, your mind and body are going to scream out, regardless of whether you're picking up a weight for the first time or doing it for the thousandth time. The good news is, it will get easier. Human beings are most comfortable with routine, not change, and predictably, you're not going to want to hear a lot of the things your body is going to tell you in the first eight weeks. So get ready to crack the whip a bit. Your challenge in the beginning might be trying to finish workouts. As a result, your sessions might take a little longer at first, and you might need longer rest periods in between. Just try not to be too hard on yourself during the transition. Instead, make sure that you're completing your reps and getting your workouts done. If you do that, you'll start learning to listen to your body and hearing what it's saying. Do *that*, and you'll gain an invaluable skill that will pay off at every step of your Evolution.

When I started with Ron, I had developed some bad habits. I had gotten into a routine in which I had upped the weights and slacked off on my form to where I wasn't fully firing off my muscle fibers. So he gave me some simple drills to help me refocus the mind–muscle connection. Try these first in a mirror; then remember the sensation for later.

Trick 1: When sitting—it can be anywhere from the office to a movie theater—focus on contracting your abs (abdominal muscles). Try to squeeze the lower ones separate from the upper. Focus on squeezing and holding, as well as breathing. This skill will be important for all ab work.

Trick 2: When you bring your arms together—such as when sitting at a desk or during a casual conversation—try to squeeze your chest muscles. Bring your hands together and press your palms into each other and feel your pectoral muscles. Switch from upper to lower if you can. It might seem bizarre, but no one will be able to notice (until you're extremely muscular), and these techniques will pay off when you're doing exercises like the bench press.

PHASE 2: INTEGRATE (WEEKS 3–4)

Now that you've adapted through repetition and have learned to activate your muscles, your body is going to start responding more forcefully. You might begin to really enjoy your workouts and exert more than you could before. By this time, you'll have a better understanding of how your body deals with eating healthy (which you'll learn in chapter 7) and reacts to being pushed. Things that were baffling and frustrating before are going to start clicking.

The great part of the second phase is that you're going to start seeing more dramatic results, which, in turn, is going to help big-time with motivation. While most people think that the biggest changes happen in the beginning, that's true only for strength and coordination. Yes, you can make some pretty big changes early on. And you'll notice a visible transformation. But once you become stronger and can activate your muscles, *that's* when you'll really start seeing big changes, because your body will become equipped to take on more. That is exactly why it's called *training*. Through a very systematic and well-thought-out process, you are in essence training your body to adapt to harsher environments/stimulus.

During this phase, we'll start integrating more complex mechanisms directly into the training, such as the "pre-exhaust," where you isolate and fatigue your muscles, and then blast the major muscle groups with a multimuscle compound approach. For example, you might find a chest flye followed by a press. A brutal and effective combination utilized by successful body builders for more than fifty years.

Things are going to start getting really fun! And when I say "fun," I of course mean *grueling* . . .

PHASE 3: IGNITE (WEEKS 5–6)

These final two weeks are built on the mold of the old strongman-style workouts. It's like taking a time machine back to a day when men looked like men and trained liked animals. These workouts are used currently by some of the great minds behind the sport of Cross-Fit who have created a hybrid utilizing bodybuilding and powerlifting techniques.

During the "ignite" phase, your body is going to hate you. It's going to make you want to take more time to recover, but you're going to learn that you won't be able to recover significantly enough to justify the rest during those tiny breaks. You will come to realize that you will be better served to just power through.

The point of the advanced phase is to push your body to the limit; you're moving more weight in less time and increasing your overall work capacity. In the end, your ability to do more work in less time is what will make you more efficient, and your physique will have no choice but to follow.

Bear in mind that *more* isn't always best in the gym—*smarter* is best. Trust me. I meet plenty of guys who want to seem tough by talking my ear off about their three- to four-hour training sessions, and I zone out. I could give them a three-*minute* workout that would leave them balled up in the fetal position on the ground. Show me how hard you can push, not how long you can push. We know better now, and the name of the game is intensity.

"Lifting weights" is a misnomer. A better way to think about your time in the gym is *squeezing your muscles with resistance.* The weights that you use merely give you resistance to make the process of squeezing harder. The weights are an apparatus. You could do the same with a rock or a sandbag. Your muscles don't know the difference; they just know resistance.

Therefore, your job is *first* to teach your muscles how to engage so that they can contract and grow. That is what's going to cause your physical transformation.

Lifting isn't just simply picking up a weight and putting it down. Make sure that your form is so good that your muscles have no choice but to respond. My goal is to help you take the greatest advantage of every exercise you perform and help you avoid the common mistakes that most people make in the gym.

SQUAT

DO'S AND DON'TS

DO be wide enough in your stance.

DON'T be on the balls of your feet and do sink into your heels.

DON'T lean too far forward with your upper body.

DO take a deep belly breath to fill your core with air as you lower.

DO push your knees out as you lower into a squat.

WHERE YOU SHOULD FEEL IT

- Lateral quads   - Glutes   - Hamstrings

BENCH

DO'S AND DON'TS

DO keep your shoulder blades back and locked together throughout the exercise.

DON'T allow your elbows to flare out wide.

DO drive your elbows down and into your rib cage.

DO grab the bar tightly and try to rip it apart with your hands to create tension.

DO keep your feet locked on the floor and slightly behind your knees.

WHERE YOU SHOULD FEEL IT

■ Pectoralis major ■ Pectoralis minor ■ Triceps

DEAD LIFT

DO'S AND DON'TS

DO bend at your hips.

DON'T round your upper back.

DO create tension in your upper back.

DO take a deep breath before pulling.

DO get a strong enough grip before the pull.

DON'T forget to keep your shoulders and elbows locked in place.

DO finish the move by thrusting your hips and squeezing your glutes.

WHERE YOU SHOULD FEEL IT

■ Hamstrings ■ Glutes ■ Quads

OVERHEAD PRESS

DO'S AND DON'TS

DO keep tension on your shoulders throughout the entire range of motion.

DON'T completely lock out your elbows at the top of the movement.

DO squeeze your glutes as you press the weight overhead to support your lower back.

DO use flexibility work to help with range of motion.

DON'T lean back or arch your back to create leverage.

DO keep your shoulder blades locked down and back for stability.

DO keep your core tight for stability.

WHERE YOU SHOULD FEEL IT

- Shoulders

ROW

DO'S AND DON'TS

DO use a tight grip.

DO allow for a natural slight arch to occur in your lower back.

DON'T round your upper back during the lift.

DON'T pull or twist your upper body to create momentum.

DO drive your elbows up and back into your rib cage.

DON'T pull with your biceps instead of your back.

DO bend at your hips and set your core for stability.

WHERE YOU SHOULD FEEL IT

- Upper back - Traps - Lats - Biceps

THE BIGGER PICTURE

Training is a means to put your health, your life, and the ability to control your destiny in your own hands. The harder you train, the better your quality of life will be. One workout at a time, one body part at a time . . . one round, one set, one rep, one positive, one negative . . . one breath, in and out. Focus! Concentrate on making each one better than the last. Now put your shoes on: It's time!

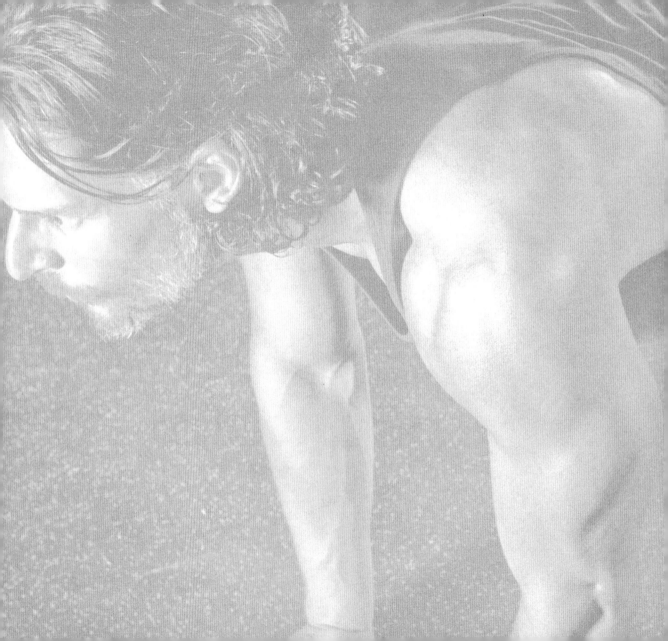

CHAPTER 6

The
Evolution
6-Week
Transformation

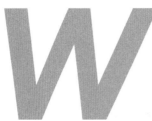

hat follows is the original "Werewolf Workout," affectionately named by my trainer Ron and me. It's the exact program I used to transform initially for my role as the often shirtless werewolf Alcide Herveaux on *True Blood*. Ron had the daunting task of creating a plan that would make me look superhuman: half man, half wolf. It was about blending aspects of muscle and strength, with a fat-loss protocol that would reveal separation between all of my muscles.

Nothing about this program is easy, but the template below is simple to follow. You should of course talk to your physician before starting this or any new fitness or diet regimen, and it's often helpful to have a professional trainer guide you. But for the most part, anyone can do this program, learn from it, and replicate it. The real difficulty lies in the mental side of the program. Staying *consistent*. Making the personal decision to spend six days a week in the gym working harder than you've ever worked before. Remember, it's not about going through the motions. It's about learning to increase the intensity of everything you do, so that every single set and every single rep is more effective.

This is the plan that can take you to the next level and show you just what you're really capable of achieving. Remind yourself of that when it gets tough. Envision what you can become, once the work is put in. To paraphrase the Godfather of Soul, James Brown, you gotta pay the cost to be the boss. Consider this your down payment.

THE EVOLUTION 6-WEEK TRANSFORMATION

Read each week carefully to understand the plan and exactly how it should be performed. Each workout begins with a warm-up, followed by a prescriptive plan of exercise, reps, sets, and rest periods. All exercise descriptions can be found in chapter 11.

THE DYNAMIC WARM-UP

Before every workout you'll notice a mention of a dynamic warm-up. This is required before you start any workout and might be the real secret to seeing results. Why, you ask? A "cold" muscle is inefficient. It doesn't transfer maximal energy and isn't as elastic, meaning you have less range of motion and are more susceptible to injury. The warm-up helps prepare your muscles for the workout, allows for maximum muscle contraction, and significantly *decreases* the likelihood that you'll get hurt. And when it comes to making an *Evolution* transformation, staying healthy is the top priority.

Each workout should begin with the following movements. Perform one exercise after another with just your body weight and with as little rest as possible. Again, all descriptions will also be found in chapter 11.

One-leg Lunges: 20 reps per leg

Squats: 15 reps

Push-ups: 15 reps

Side-to-side jumps: 30 seconds

Front-to-back jumps: 30 seconds

WEEK 1: 3-DAY SPLIT: *(1) Chest and Back, (2) Legs and Triceps, (3) Shoulders and Biceps—6 Days On, 1 Off*

MONDAY: CHEST AND BACK

- Dynamic Warm-Up

- Circuit 1: This couplet set is performed with little or no rest between each set until both exercises are completed. In order to perform circuits correctly, progress through all the exercises and then rest. For example, the first set will consist of 20 reps of bench press followed by 20 reps of lat pull-downs, and then you'll rest. After that, you'll do 15 reps of bench press followed by 15 reps of lat pull-downs—and then another period of rest. You'll complete this for all sets of each exercise, rest, and then move on to the next circuit. This is the strategy you'll apply for all circuits, unless instructed otherwise.

  Barbell Bench Press: sets of 20, 15, 12, 10, 5, 8, and 16 reps; weight will be moderate, so that you can get all of the reps with good form.

  Lat Pull-Down with Wide Pronated Grip: sets of 20, 15 ,12, 10, 5, 8, and 16 reps; weight will be moderate, so that you can get all of the reps with good form.

  Rest 1 minute and then repeat circuit, performing a total of 7 sets each of bench press and lat pull-downs.

- Circuit 2: This couplet set is performed with little or no rest between each set until both exercises are completed.

  Dumbbell Incline Press: 12 to 15 reps; weight will be light to moderate, so that you can get all of the reps with good form and a good isometric contraction at the peak.

  One-Arm Dumbbell Row with Neutral Grip: 10 to 12 reps each arm.

  Rest 1 minute and then repeat circuit. Do this 4 times. Push yourself to stay at the same weight, or slightly increase the weight on each set.

- Circuit 3: This couplet set is performed with little or no rest between each set until both exercises are completed.

   Pec Deck: 10 reps; weight will be moderate, so that you can get all of the reps with good form.

   Low Row with Narrow Neutral Grip: 10 reps; weight will be moderate, so that you can get all of the reps with good form.

   Rest 1 minute and then repeat circuit. Do this 4 times. Push yourself to stay at the same weight, or slightly increase the weight on each set.

TUESDAY: LEGS AND TRICEPS

- Dynamic Warm-Up

- Circuit 1: This couplet set is performed with little or no rest between each set until both exercises are completed.

   Barbell Back Squat: sets of 20, 15, 12, 10, 5, 8, and 16 reps; weight will be moderate, so that you can get all of the reps with good form.

   V-Bar Triceps Extension: sets of 20, 15 ,12, 10, 5, 8, and 16 reps; weight will be moderate, so that you can get all of the reps with good form.

   Rest 1 minute and then repeat circuit until done.

- Circuit 2: This couplet set is performed with little or no rest between each set until both exercises are completed.

   Leg Curl: 12 to 15 reps; weight will be light to moderate, so that you can get all of the reps with good form and a good isometric contraction at the peak.

   One-Arm Dumbbell Lying Triceps Extension: 10 to 12 reps each arm.

   Rest 1 minute and then repeat circuit. Do this 4 times. Push yourself to stay at the same weight, or slightly increase the weight on each set.

- Circuit 3: This couplet set is performed with little or no rest between each set until both exercises are completed.

> **Dumbbell or Kettlebell Goblet Squat:** 10 reps; weight will be moderate, so that you can get all of the reps with good form.

> **Two-Arm, One-Dumbbell Overhead Triceps Extension:** 15 reps; weight will be moderate, so that you can get all of the reps with good form.

> Rest 1 minute and then repeat circuit. Do this 4 times. Push yourself to stay at the same weight, or slightly increase the weight on each set.

WEDNESDAY: DELTOIDS AND BICEPS

- Dynamic Warm-Up
- Circuit 1: This couplet set is performed with little or no rest between each set until both exercises are completed.

> **Seated Dumbbell Overhead Press:** sets of 20, 15 ,12, 10, 5, 8, and 16 reps; weight will be moderate, so that you can get all of the reps with good form.

> **Seated Dumbbell Two-Arm Curl:** sets of 20, 15 ,12, 10, 5, 8, and 16 reps; weight will be moderate, so that you can get all of the reps with good form.

> Rest 1 minute and then repeat circuit until done.

- Circuit 2: This couplet set is performed with little or no rest between each set until both exercises are completed.

> **Plate Front Raise:** 12 to 15 reps; weight will be light to moderate, so that you can get all of the reps with good form.

> **Standing Barbell Curl:** 10 to 12 reps each arm.

> Rest 1 minute and then repeat circuit. Do this 4 times. Push yourself to stay at the same weight, or slightly increase the weight on each set.

- Circuit 3: This couplet set is performed with little or no rest between each set until both exercises are completed.

    Dumbbell Lateral Raise: 12 reps; weight will be moderate, so that you can get all of the reps with good form.

    Dumbbell Hammer Curl: 12 reps; weight will be moderate, so that you can get all of the reps with good form.

    Rest 1 minute and then repeat circuit. Do this 4 times. Push yourself to stay at the same weight, or slightly increase the weight on each set.

THURSDAY: CHEST AND BACK

- Dynamic Warm-Up
- Circuit 1: This couplet set is performed with little or no rest between each set until both exercises are completed.

    Dumbbell Flye: sets of 15, 12, 10, 10, and 10 reps; weight will be moderate, so that you can get all of the reps with good form.

    Two-Arm Bent-Over Dumbbell Row with Neutral Grip: sets of 15, 12, 10, 10, and 10 reps; weight will be moderate, so that you can get all of the reps with good form.

    Rest 1 minute and then repeat circuit until done.

- Circuit 2: This couplet set is performed with little or no rest between each set until both exercises are completed.

    Close-Grip Barbell Bench Press: 10 to 12 reps; weight will be light to moderate, so that you can get all of the reps with good form. The close grip will be 12 inches between the hands.

    Lat Pull-Down with Narrow Supinated Grip: 10 to 12 reps.

    Rest 1 minute and then repeat circuit. Do this 4 times. Push yourself to stay at the same weight, or slightly increase the weight on each set.

- Circuit 3: This couplet set is performed with little or no rest between each set until both exercises are completed.

   Bar Dip: AMRAP (as many reps as possible); shoulder must go below height of elbow and must lock out arms on each rep to count.

   Low Row with Narrow Supinated Grip: 10 to 12 reps; weight will be moderate, so that you can get all of the reps with good form.

   Rest 1 minute and then repeat circuit. Do this 4 times. Push yourself to stay at the same weight, or slightly increase the weight on each set.

FRIDAY: LEGS AND TRICEPS

- Dynamic Warm-Up
- Circuit 1: This couplet set is performed with little or no rest between each set until both exercises are completed.

   Reverse Lunge: sets of 15, 12, 10, 10, and 10 reps; weight will be moderate, so that you can get all of the reps with good form.

   Straight-Bar Triceps Extension: sets of 15, 12, 10, 10, and 10 reps; weight will be moderate, so that you can get all of the reps with good form.

   Rest 1 minute and then repeat circuit until done.

- Circuit 2: This couplet set is performed with little or no rest between each set until both exercises are completed.

   Leg Extension: 10 to 12 reps; weight will be light to moderate, so that you can get all of the reps with good form and a good isometric contraction at the peak.

   French Press: 10 to 12 reps.

   Rest 1 minute and then repeat circuit. Do this 4 times. Push yourself to stay at the same weight, or slightly increase the weight on each set.

- Circuit 3: This couplet set is performed with little or no rest between each set until both exercises are completed.

  Barbell Front Squat: 10 reps; weight will be moderate, so that you can get all of the reps with good form.

  Rope Triceps Extension in Front of Body: 15 reps; weight will be moderate, so that you can get all of the reps with good form.

  Rest 1 minute and then repeat circuit. Do this 4 times. Push yourself to stay at the same weight, or slightly increase the weight on each set.

SATURDAY: DELTOIDS AND BICEPS

- Dynamic Warm-Up

- Circuit 1: This couplet set is performed with little or no rest between each set until both exercises are completed.

  Barbell Upright Row: sets of 15, 12, 10, 10, and 10 reps; weight will be moderate, so that you can get all of the reps with good form.

  Triple Dumbbell Curl: sets of 15, 12, 10, 10, and 10 reps; weight will be moderate, so that you can get all of the reps with good form.

  Rest 1 minute and then repeat circuit until done.

- Circuit 2: This couplet set is performed with little or no rest between each set until both exercises are completed.

  Seated Dumbbell Overhead Press: 10 to 12 reps; weight will be light to moderate, so that you can get all of the reps with good form.

  Straight-Bar Cable Curl: 10 to 12 reps.

  Rest 1 minute and then repeat circuit. Do this 4 times. Push yourself to stay at the same weight, or slightly increase the weight on each set.

- Circuit 3: This couplet set is performed with little or no rest between each set until both exercises are completed.

> **Dumbbell Rotating Lateral Raise:** 12 reps; weight will be moderate, so that you can get all of the reps with good form.

> **Dumbbell Alternating Curl:** 20 reps, 10 each arm; weight will be moderate, so that you can get all of the reps with good form.

> Rest 1 minute and then repeat circuit. Do this 4 times. Push yourself to stay at the same weight, or slightly increase the weight on each set.

SUNDAY: OFF

WEEK 2: 3-DAY SPLIT: *(1) Chest and Back, (2) Legs and Triceps, (3) Shoulders and Biceps—6 Days On, 1 Off*

MONDAY: CHEST AND BACK

- Dynamic Warm-Up
- Do the same workout from week 1, except cut down the rest time to 50 seconds.
- After the workout: Go directly into low- to medium-intensity cardio. Can be any variant that you like (stairs, treadmill, rower, jogging outside), but you must keep a consistent pace, with your heart rate in the 120-to-130 (beats per minute) range for at least 20 minutes.

TUESDAY: LEGS AND TRICEPS

- Dynamic Warm-Up
- Do the same workout from week 1, except cut down the rest time to 50 seconds.

WEDNESDAY: DELTOIDS AND BICEPS

- Dynamic Warm-Up

- Do an Ab Program. (See page 124.)

- Do the same workout from week 1, except cut down the rest time to 50 seconds.

THURSDAY: CHEST AND BACK

- Dynamic Warm-Up

- Do the same workout from week 1, except cut down the rest time to 50 seconds.

- After the workout: Go directly into low- to medium-intensity cardio. Can be any variant that you like (stairs, treadmill, rower, jogging outside), but you must keep a consistent pace, with your heart rate in the 120-to-130 range for at least 20 minutes.

FRIDAY: LEGS AND TRICEPS

- Dynamic Warm-Up

- Do the same workout from week 1, except cut down the rest time to 50 seconds.

SATURDAY: DELTOIDS AND BICEPS

- Dynamic Warm-Up

- Do an Ab Program. (See page 124.) Do the same workout from week 1, except cut down the rest time to 50 seconds.

SUNDAY: OFF

WEEK 3: 3-DAY SPLIT: *(1) Chest and Back, (2) Legs and Triceps, (3) Shoulders and Biceps—6 Days On, 1 Off*

MONDAY: CHEST AND BACK

- Dynamic Warm-Up

- Circuit 1: This triplet set is performed with little or no rest between each set until all three exercises are completed.

    Barbell Incline Press: 15 reps; weight will be moderate, so that you can get all of the reps with good form.

    Pull-Up with Wide Pronated Grip: 4 to 10 reps; even if you can only do 1, work on getting the form down.

    Lat Pull-Down with Wide Pronated Grip: 12 to 15 reps; weight will be moderate, so that you can get all of the reps with good form.

    Rest 1 minute and then repeat circuit. Do this 4 times. Push yourself to stay at the same weight, or slightly increase the weight on each set.

- Circuit 2: This triplet set is performed with little or no rest between each set until all three exercises are completed.

    Cable Chest Flye: 12 to 15 reps; weight will be light to moderate, so that you can get all of the reps with good form and a good isometric contraction at the peak.

    Push-Up: 15 reps; drop down immediately after the last flye rep.

    Low Row with Narrow Neutral Grip: 12 to 15 reps; weight will be moderate, so that you can get all of the reps with good form.

    Rest 1 minute and then repeat circuit. Do this 4 times. Push yourself to stay at the same weight, or slightly increase the weight on each set.

- Circuit 3: This couplet set is performed with little or no rest between each set until both exercises are completed.

  Dumbbell Bench Press: 12 reps; weight will be moderate, so that you can get all of the reps with good form.

  Bent-Over Barbell Row with Wide Pronated Grip: 10 reps; weight will be moderate, so that you can get all of the reps with good form.

  Rest 1 minute and then repeat circuit. Do this 4 times. Push yourself to stay at the same weight, or slightly increase the weight on each set.

- After the workout: Go directly into low- to medium-intensity cardio. Can be any variant that you like (stairs, treadmill, rower, jogging outside), but you must keep a consistent pace, with your heart rate in the 120-to-130 range for at least 20 minutes.

TUESDAY: LEGS AND TRICEPS

- Dynamic Warm-Up

- Do an Ab Program. (See page 124.)

- Circuit 1: This triplet set is performed with little or no rest between each set until all three exercises are completed.

  Barbell Back Squat: 15 reps; weight will be moderate, so that you can get all of the reps with good form.

  EZ-Bar Nosebuster: 12 reps; weight will be moderate, so that you can get all of the reps with good form.

  EZ-Bar (or Barbell) Triceps Press with Narrow Grip: go right into it with the same weight as the Nosebuster.

  Rest 1 minute and then repeat circuit. Do this 4 times. Push yourself to stay at the same weight, or slightly increase the weight on each set.

- Circuit 2: This triplet set is performed with little or no rest between each set until all three exercises are completed.

  Bulgarian Split Squat: 12 to 15 reps; weight will be light to moderate, so that you can get all of the reps with good form.

  Rope Triceps Extension—Overhead: 12 reps; weight will be light to moderate, so that you can get all of the reps with good form.

  Rope Triceps Extension in Front of Body: 12 reps; weight will be light to moderate, so that you can get all of the reps with good form.

  Rest 1 minute and then repeat circuit. Do this 4 times. Push yourself to stay at the same weight, or slightly increase the weight on each set.

- Circuit 3: This couplet set is performed with little or no rest between each set until both exercises are completed.

  Dumbbell Bench Step-Up: 20 reps, 10 each leg; weight will be light, so that you can get all of the reps with good form.

  Bench Dip: 20 reps; really pay attention to form on this one.

  Rest 1 minute and then repeat circuit. Do this 4 times. Push yourself and stay at the same dumbbell weight on each set.

WEDNESDAY: SHOULDERS AND BICEPS

- Dynamic Warm-Up

- Circuit 1: This triplet set is performed with little or no rest between each set until all three exercises are completed.

  Standing Military Press: 10 reps; weight will be moderate, so that you can get all of the reps with good form.

  (Light) Standing Military Press: 12 reps; drop the weight from the first set by 40 percent. Try to have the barbell set up so that you can pause only long enough to strip the desired weight off each end of the bar and then get back in it. This should take only 10 to 15 seconds.

Standing Barbell Curl: 10 to 12 reps; use the same bar and either use the same weight as the last Military Press or add a little more. Make this transition fast! Under 20 seconds.

Rest 1 minute and then repeat circuit. Do this 4 times. Push yourself to stay at the same weight, or slightly increase the weight on each set.

- Circuit 2: This couplet set is performed with little or no rest between each set until both exercises are completed.

   Cable One-Arm Lateral Raise: 12 to 15 reps; weight will be light to moderate, so that you can get all of the reps with good form and a good isometric contraction at the peak.

   Dumbbell Alternating Curl with Twist: 20 reps, 10 each arm.

   Rest 1 minute and then repeat circuit. Do this 4 times. Push yourself to stay at the same weight.

- Circuit 3: This triplet set is performed with little or no rest between each set until all three exercises are completed.

   Dumbbell Front Raise: 10 reps; weight will be light, so that you can get all of the reps with good form.

   Dumbbell Rear-Deltoid Raise: use the same dumbbells from the Front Raise; go right into it.

   Rope Hammer Curl (drop set): 10 reps; drop the weight and do 10 more.

   Rest 1 minute and then repeat circuit. Do this 4 times. Push yourself to stay at the same weight.

- After the workout: Go directly into low- to medium-intensity cardio. Can be any variant that you like (stairs, treadmill, rower, jogging outside), but you must keep a consistent pace, with your heart rate in the 120-to-130 range for at least 20 minutes.

THURSDAY: CHEST AND BACK

- Dynamic Warm-Up

- Do an Ab Program. (See page 124.)

- Circuit 1: This triplet set is performed with little or no rest between each set until all three exercises are completed.

    Barbell Bench Press: 15 reps; weight will be moderate, so that you can get all of the reps with good form.

    Chin-Up with Narrow Supinated Grip: 4 to 10 reps; even if you can only do 1, work on getting the form down.

    Lat Pull-Down with Narrow Neutral Grip: 12 to 15 reps; weight will be moderate, so that you can get all of the reps with good form.

    Rest 1 minute and then repeat circuit. Do this 4 times. Push yourself to stay at the same weight, or slightly increase the weight on each set.

- Circuit 2: This triplet set is performed with little or no rest between each set until all three exercises are completed.

    Pec Deck: 12 to 15 reps; weight will be light to moderate, so that you can get all of the reps with good form and a good isometric contraction at the peak.

    Bar Dip: 15 reps; if you cannot do Bar Dips, substitute Push-Ups.

    One-Arm Dumbbell Row with Supinated Grip: 12 reps each arm; weight will be moderate to heavy, but make sure that you can get all of the reps with good form.

    Rest 1 minute and then repeat circuit. Do this 4 times. Push yourself to stay at the same weight, or slightly increase the weight on each set.

- Circuit 3: This triplet set is performed with little or no rest between each set until all three exercises are completed.

    Bench Plyo Push-Up: 10 reps.

    Bench Push-Up: 10 reps.

Low Row with Wide Pronated Grip: 10 reps; weight will be moderate, so that you can get all of the reps with good form.

Rest 1 minute and then repeat circuit. Do this 4 times. Push yourself to stay at the same weight, or slightly increase the weight on each set.

FRIDAY: LEGS AND TRICEPS

- Dynamic Warm-Up
- Circuit 1: This couplet set is performed with little or no rest between each set until both exercises are completed.

    Dead Lift: 15 reps; weight will be moderate, so that you can get all of the reps with good form.

    Lying J Press: 12 reps; weight will be moderate, so that you can get all of the reps with good form.

    Rest 1 minute and then repeat circuit. Do this 4 times. Push yourself to stay at the same weight, or slightly increase the weight on each set.

- Circuit 2: This triplet set is performed with little or no rest between each set until all three exercises are completed.

    Dumbbell Walking Lunge: 15 steps with each leg; weight will be light to moderate, so that you can get all of the reps with good form.

    (Heavy) V-Bar Triceps Extension: 10 reps; weight will be heavy, but get all of the reps with good form.

    V-Bar Triceps Extension: 10 reps; weight will be moderate, but get all of the reps with good form.

    Rest 1 minute and then repeat circuit. Do this 4 times. Push yourself to stay at the same weight, or slightly increase the weight on each set.

- Circuit 3: This triplet set is performed with little or no rest between each set until all three exercises are completed.

Leg Extension: 12 reps; weight will be moderate, so that you can get all of the reps with good form.

Leg Curl: 12 reps; weight will be moderate, so that you can get all of the reps with good form.

One-Arm Dumbbell Lying Triceps Extension: 12 reps each arm.

Rest 1 minute and then repeat circuit. Do this 4 times. Push yourself to stay at the same weight on each set.

- After the workout: Go directly into low- to medium-intensity cardio. Can be any variant that you like (stairs, treadmill, rower, jogging outside), but you must keep a consistent pace, with your heart rate in the 120-to-130 range for at least 20 minutes.

SATURDAY: SHOULDERS AND BICEPS

- Dynamic Warm-Up

- Do an Ab Program. (See page 124.)

- Circuit 1: This triplet set is performed with little or no rest between each set until all three exercises are completed.

    Neutral-Grip Machine Overhead Press: 12 reps; weight will be moderate, so that you can get all of the reps with good form.

    Dumbbell Alternating Curl: 10 reps each arm; weight will be moderate, so that you can get all of the reps with good form. Drop set into

    (Light) Dumbbell Alternating Curl: 10 reps; drop the weight from the first set by 10 to 15 pounds per dumbbell and then go right into this set.

    Rest 1 minute and then repeat circuit. Do this 4 times. Push yourself to stay at the same weight.

- Circuit 2: This triplet set is performed with little or no rest between each set until all three exercises are completed.

Dumbbell Lateral Raise: 12 reps; weight will be light to moderate, so that you can get all of the reps with good form and a good isometric contraction at the peak.

Seated Arnold Press: 12 reps; use the same dumbbells as the lateral raise and go right into it. Adjust reps to do as many as you can with good form up to 20.

EZ-Bar Curl with Outside Grip: 15 reps.

Rest 1 minute and then repeat circuit. Do this 4 times. Push yourself to stay at the same weight.

- Circuit 3: This triplet set is performed with little or no rest between each set until all three exercises are completed.

    Cable One-Arm Bent-Over Rear-Deltoid Raise: 10 reps each; weight will be light, so that you can get all of the reps with good form.

    Preacher Curl: 10 reps; weight will be moderate, so that you can get all of the reps with good form,

    Preacher Curl Pulse: 10 reps, performed right after full-range sets with same weight.

    Rest 1 minute and then repeat circuit. Do this 4 times. Push yourself to stay at the same weight.

SUNDAY: OFF

WEEK 4: 3-DAY SPLIT: *(1) Chest and Back, (2) Legs and Triceps, (3) Shoulders and Biceps—6 Days On, 1 Off*

- The workouts are the same as week 3, with these exceptions:
- All rest times between couplet and triplet sets cut down to 50 seconds;
- 20 minutes of cardio after every workout (including ab days).

MONDAY: CHEST AND BACK

- Dynamic Warm-Up

- Do the same workout from week 3, except cut down the rest time to 50 seconds.

- After the workout: Go directly into low- to medium-intensity cardio. Can be any variant that you like (stairs, treadmill, rower, jogging outside), but you must keep a consistent pace, with your heart rate in the 120-to-130 range for at least 20 minutes.

TUESDAY: LEGS AND TRICEPS

- Dynamic Warm-Up

- Do an Ab Program. (See page 124.)

- Do the same workout from week 3, except cut down the rest time to 50 seconds.

- After the workout: Go directly into low- to medium-intensity cardio. Can be any variant that you like (stairs, treadmill, rower, jogging outside), but you must keep a consistent pace, with your heart rate in the 120-to-130 range for at least 20 minutes.

WEDNESDAY: DELTOIDS AND BICEPS

- Dynamic Warm-Up

- Do the same workout from week 3, except cut down the rest time to 50 seconds.

- After the workout: Go directly into low- to medium-intensity cardio. Can be any variant that you like (stairs, treadmill, rower, jogging outside), but you must keep a consistent pace, with your heart rate in the 120-to-130 range for at least 20 minutes.

THURSDAY: CHEST AND BACK

- Dynamic Warm-Up

- Do an Ab Program. (See page 122.)

- Do the same workout from week 3, except cut down the rest time to 50 seconds.

- After the workout: Go directly into 20 minutes of low- to medium-intensity cardio. Can be any variant that you like (stairs, treadmill, rower, jogging outside), but you must keep a consistent pace, with your heart rate in the 120-to-130 range for at least 20 minutes.

FRIDAY: LEGS AND TRICEPS

- Dynamic Warm-Up

- Do the same workout from week 3, except cut down the rest time to 50 seconds.

- After the workout: Go directly into 20 minutes of low- to medium-intensity cardio. Can be any variant that you like (stairs, treadmill, rower, jogging outside), but you must keep a consistent pace, with your heart rate in the 120-to-130 range for at least 20 minutes.

SATURDAY: DELTOIDS AND BICEPS

- Dynamic Warm-Up

- Do an Ab Program. (See page 124.)

- Do the same workout from week 3, except cut down the rest time to 50 seconds.

- After the workout: Go directly into low- to medium-intensity cardio. Can be any variant that you like (stairs, treadmill, rower, jogging outside), but you must keep a consistent pace, with your heart rate in the 120-to-130 range for at least 20 minutes.

SUNDAY: OFF

WEEK 5: 3-DAY SPLIT: *(1) Chest and Back, (2) Legs and Triceps, (3) Shoulders and Biceps—6 Days On, 1 Off*

MONDAY: CHEST AND BACK

Workout 1 (Preferably First Thing in the Morning on an Empty Stomach)

- 30 to 45 minutes of low- to medium-intensity cardio. Can be any variant that you like (stairs, treadmill, rower, jogging outside), but you must keep a consistent pace, with your heart rate in the 120-to-130 range.

Workout 2 (Some Other Time During the Day)

- Dynamic Warm-Up

- Do an Ab Program. (See page 124.)

- Circuit 1: This quartet of exercises (oftentimes referred to as a "giant set") is performed with little or no rest between each set until all four exercises are completed.

    Dumbbell Flye: 10 reps; weight will be moderate, so that you can get all of the reps with good form.

    Dumbbell Bench Press: 10 reps; weight will be moderate, so that you can get all of the reps with good form.

    Push-Up: 10 reps.

    Lat Pull-Down with Wide Neutral Grip: 12 reps.

    Rest 1 minute and then repeat circuit. Do this 4 times. Push yourself to stay at the same weight, or slightly increase the weight on each set.

- Circuit 2: This couplet set is performed with little or no rest between each set until both exercises are completed.

    Low Row with Narrow Neutral Grip (drop set): 5 reps; lower the weight for 10 reps and then lower the weight again for 15 reps.

    Barbell Incline Press: 12 reps.

Rest 1 minute and then repeat circuit. Do this 4 times. Push your-self to stay at the same weight, or slightly increase the weight on each set.

- Circuit 3: This couplet set is performed with little or no rest between each set until both exercises are completed.

  Bar Dip: 12 reps.

  Bent-Over Supinated Low Cable Row: 12 reps; weight will be moderate, so that you can get all of the reps with good form.

  Rest 1 minute and then repeat circuit. Do this 4 times. Push your-self to stay at the same weight, or slightly increase the weight on each set.

- Circuit 4: This couplet set is performed with little or no rest between each set until both exercises are completed.

  Narrow-Grip Bench Push-Up: 12 reps.

  Barbell Pull-Over: 12 reps; weight will be moderate, so that you can get all of the reps with good form.

  Rest 1 minute and then repeat circuit. Do this 4 times. Push your-self to stay at the same weight, or slightly increase the weight on each set.

TUESDAY: LEGS AND TRICEPS

Workout 1 (Preferably First Thing in the Morning on an Empty Stomach)

- 30 to 45 minutes of low- to medium-intensity cardio. Can be any variant that you like (stairs, treadmill, rower, jogging outside), but you must keep a consistent pace, with your heart rate in the 120-to-130 range.

Workout 2 (Some Other Time During the Day)

- Dynamic Warm-Up

- Circuit 1: This giant set is performed with little or no rest between each set until all four exercises are completed.

    Barbell Back Squat: 10 reps; weight will be moderate, so that you can get all of the reps with good form.

    Plyo Squat Jump: 10 reps.

    Body-Weight Squat: 10 reps.

    Diamond Push-Up: 15 reps.

    Rest 1 minute and then repeat circuit. Do this 4 times. Push yourself to stay at the same weight, or slightly increase the weight on each set.

- Circuit 2: This triplet set is performed with little or no rest between each set until all three exercises are completed.

    One-Leg Leg Curl: 12 reps; start with the left leg and then go directly into the Lunge, also with the left leg. Then repeat the Leg Curl with the right leg and the Lunge, also with the right leg. When you've finished these 2 exercises go to the V-Bar Triceps Extension.

    One-Leg Lunge: 12 reps each.

    V-Bar Triceps Extension (triple drop set): 10 reps; lower the weight for 10 reps and then lower the weight again for 10 reps.

    Rest 1 minute and then repeat circuit. Do this 4 times. Push yourself to stay at the same weight, or slightly increase the weight on each set.

- Circuit 3: This couplet set is performed with little or no rest between each set until both exercises are completed.

    Box or Bench Jump: 15 reps; stand up all the way each time on the Jump.

    Bench Dip: 15 reps.

Rest 1 minute and then repeat circuit. Do this 4 times. Push yourself to stay at the same weight, or slightly increase the weight on each set.

- Circuit 4: This couplet set is performed with little or no rest between each set until both exercises are completed.

    One-Leg Bench Bridge: 15 reps each leg.

    Burpee: 15 reps.

    Rest 1 minute and then repeat circuit. Do this 4 times. Push yourself to stay at the same weight, or slightly increase the weight on each set.

WEDNESDAY: DELTOIDS AND BICEPS

Workout 1 (Preferably First Thing in the Morning on an Empty Stomach)

- 30 to 45 minutes of low- to medium-intensity cardio. Can be any variant that you like (stairs, treadmill, rower, jogging outside), but you must keep a consistent pace, with your heart rate in the 120-to-130 range.

Workout 2 (Some Other Time During the Day)

- Dynamic Warm-Up

- Do an Ab Program. (See page 124.)

- Circuit 1: This couplet set is performed with little or no rest between each set until both exercises are completed.

    Seated Military Press (drop set): 5 reps; lower the weight for 10 reps and then lower the weight again for 15 reps.

    EZ-Bar Curl with Narrow Grip and with Outside Grip: 12 reps; switch grips from outside to inside and do 2 sets each.

    Rest 1 minute and then repeat circuit. Do this 4 times. Push yourself to stay at the same weight, or slightly increase the weight on each set.

- Circuit 2: This couplet set is performed with little or no rest between each set until both exercises are completed.

  Seated Rear-Deltoid Bent-Over Dumbbell Reverse Flye (drop set): 12 reps; lower the weight for 12 reps.

  Dumbbell Alternating Curl with Twist (drop set): 6 reps each; lower the weight for 8 reps each and then lower the weight again for 10 reps each.

  Rest 1 minute and then repeat circuit. Do this 4 times. Push yourself to stay at the same weight, or slightly increase the weight on each set.

- Circuit 3: This couplet set is performed with little or no rest between each set until both exercises are completed.

  Rope Front Raise: 12 reps.

  Rope Hammer Curl: 12 reps; weight will be moderate, so that you can get all of the reps with good form.

  Rest 1 minute and then repeat circuit. Do this 4 times. Push yourself to stay at the same weight, or slightly increase the weight on each set.

- Circuit 4: This couplet set is performed with little or no rest between each set until both exercises are completed.

  Dumbbell Lateral Raise: 12 reps.

  Triple Dumbbell Curl: 12 reps each; weight will be light, so that you can get all of the reps with good form.

  Rest 1 minute and then repeat circuit. Do this 4 times. Push yourself to stay at the same weight, or slightly increase the weight on each set.

THURSDAY: CHEST AND BACK

Workout 1 (Preferably First Thing in the Morning on an Empty Stomach)

- 30 to 45 minutes of low- to medium-intensity cardio. Can be any variant that you like (stairs, treadmill, rower, jogging outside), but you must keep a consistent pace, with your heart rate in the 120-to-130 range.

Workout 2 (Some Other Time During the Day)

- Dynamic Warm-Up

- Circuit 1: This couplet set is performed with little or no rest between each set until both exercises are completed.

    Lat Pull-Down with Wide Pronated Grip (drop set): 5 reps; lower the weight for 10 reps, and then lower the weight again for 15 reps.

    Push-Up: 20 reps.

    Rest 1 minute and then repeat circuit. Do this 4 times. Push yourself to stay at the same weight, or slightly increase the weight on each set.

- Circuit 2: This triplet set is performed with little or no rest between each set until all three exercises are completed.

    Barbell Bench Press (drop set): 5 reps; lower the weight for 10 reps, and then lower the weight again for 15 reps.

    Seated Dumbbell Row: 12 reps.

    Seated Dumbbell Swim and Row: 12 reps.

    Rest 1 minute and then repeat circuit. Do this 4 times. Push yourself to stay at the same weight, or slightly increase the weight on each set.

- Circuit 3: This couplet set is performed with little or no rest between each set until both exercises are completed.

Plyo Push-Up Over a Plate: 20 reps.

Standing Front-Lat Push-Down: 12 reps; weight will be moderate, so that you can get all of the reps with good form.

Rest 1 minute and then repeat circuit. Do this 4 times. Push yourself to stay at the same weight, or slightly increase the weight on each set.

- Circuit 4: This couplet set is performed with little or no rest between each set until both exercises are completed.

    Pec Deck: 12 reps.

    Lat Pull-Down with Narrow Neutral Grip: 12 reps.

    Rest 1 minute and then repeat circuit. Do this 4 times. Push yourself to stay at the same weight, or slightly increase the weight on each set.

FRIDAY: LEGS AND TRICEPS

Workout 1 (Preferably First Thing in the Morning on an Empty Stomach)

- 30 to 45 minutes of low- to medium-intensity cardio. Can be any variant that you like (stairs, treadmill, rower, jogging outside), but you must keep a consistent pace, with your heart rate in the 120-to-130 range.

Workout 2 (Some Other Time During the Day)

- Dynamic Warm-Up

- Do an Ab Program. (See page 124.)

- Circuit 1: This giant set is performed with little or no rest between each set until all four exercises are completed.

    Dumbbell Bench Step-Up: 10 reps each leg.

    Plyo Step-Up with a Jump: 10 reps each leg.

    Body-Weight Step-Up: 10 reps each leg.

    Body-Weight Nosebuster: 15 reps.

Rest 1 minute and then repeat circuit. Do this 4 times. Push yourself to stay at the same weight, or slightly increase the weight on each set.

- Circuit 2: This couplet set is performed with little or no rest between each set until both exercises are completed.

  Leg Extension (drop set): 10 reps; lower the weight for 10 reps, and then lower the weight again for 10 reps.

  Straight-Bar Triceps Extension (drop set): 10 reps; lower the weight for 10 reps, and then lower the weight again for 10 reps.

  Rest 1 minute and then repeat circuit. Do this 4 times. Push yourself to stay at the same weight, or slightly increase the weight on each set.

- Circuit 3: This couplet set is performed with little or no rest between each set until both exercises are completed.

  Traveling Squat Jump: 30 reps.

  One-Arm Cable Triceps Extension (drop set): 10 reps each arm; lower the weight for 10 reps each arm, and then lower the weight again for 10 reps each arm.

  Rest 1 minute and then repeat circuit. Do this 4 times. Push yourself to stay at the same weight, or slightly increase the weight on each set.

- Circuit 4: This couplet set is performed with little or no rest between each set until both exercises are completed.

  Bench Jump-Over: 20 reps.

  One-Arm Lying Cross-Body Dumbbell Triceps Extension: 12 reps each arm.

  Rest 1 minute and then repeat circuit. Do this 4 times. Push yourself to stay at the same weight, or slightly increase the weight on each set.

SATURDAY: DELTOIDS AND BICEPS

Workout 1 (Preferably First Thing in the Morning on an Empty Stomach)

- 30 to 45 minutes of low- to medium-intensity cardio. Can be any variant that you like (stairs, treadmill, rower, jogging outside), but you must keep a consistent pace, with your heart rate in the 120-to-130 range.

Workout 2 (Some Other Time During the Day)

- Dynamic Warm-Up
- Circuit 1: This triplet set is performed with little or no rest between each set until all three exercises are completed.

   Seated Dumbbell Overhead Press: 12 reps.

   Dumbbell Lateral Raise: 12 reps.

   Seated Dumbbell Two-Arm Curl: 12 reps.

   Rest 1 minute and then repeat circuit. Do this 4 times. Push yourself to stay at the same weight, or slightly increase the weight on each set.

- Circuit 2: This couplet set is performed with little or no rest between each set until both exercises are completed.

   Standing Military Press: 10 reps.

   Standing Barbell Curl (drop set): 7 reps; lower the weight for 7 reps, and then lower the weight again for 7 reps.

   Rest 1 minute and then repeat circuit. Do this 4 times. Push yourself to stay at the same weight, or slightly increase the weight on each set.

- Circuit 3: This couplet set is performed with little or no rest between each set until both exercises are completed.

   Dumbbell Front Raise and Lateral Raise: 10 reps.

   Reverse Curl: 12 reps; weight will be moderate, so that you can get all of the reps with good form.

Rest 1 minute and then repeat circuit. Do this 4 times. Push yourself to stay at the same weight, or slightly increase the weight on each set.

- Circuit 4: This couplet set is performed with little or no rest between each set until both exercises are completed.

   Cable Two-Arm Reverse Flye: 12 reps.

   Straight-Bar Cable Curl: 12 reps.

   Rest 1 minute and then repeat circuit. Do this 4 times. Push yourself to stay at the same weight, or slightly increase the weight on each set.

SUNDAY: OFF

WEEK 6: 3-DAY SPLIT: *(1) Chest and Back, (2) Legs and Triceps, (3) Shoulders and Biceps—6 Days On, 1 Off*

- The workouts are the same as week 5, with these exceptions:
- All rest times are cut down to 50 seconds;
- 20 minutes of cardio after every workout (including ab days).

MONDAY: CHEST AND BACK

Workout 1 (Preferably First Thing in the Morning on an Empty Stomach)

- 45 to 60 minutes of low- to medium-intensity cardio. Can be any variant that you like (stairs, treadmill, rower, jogging outside), but you must keep a consistent pace, with your heart rate in the 120-to-130 range.

Workout 2 (Some Other Time During the Day)

- Dynamic Warm-Up
- Do an Ab Program. (See page 124.)

- Do the same workout from week 5, except cut down the rest time to 50 seconds.

- After the workout: Go directly into low- to medium-intensity cardio. Can be any variant that you like (stairs, treadmill, rower, jogging outside), but you must keep a consistent pace, with your heart rate in the 120-to-130 range for at least 20 minutes.

TUESDAY: LEGS AND TRICEPS

Workout 1 (Preferably First Thing in the Morning on an Empty Stomach)

- 45 to 60 minutes of low- to medium-intensity cardio. Can be any variant that you like (stairs, treadmill, rower, jogging outside), but you must keep a consistent pace, with your heart rate in the 120-to-130 range for at least 20 minutes.

Workout 2 (Some Other Time During the Day)

- Dynamic Warm-Up

- Do the same workout from week 5, except cut down the rest time to 50 seconds.

- After the workout: Go directly into 20 minutes of low- to medium-intensity cardio. Can be any variant that you like (stairs, treadmill, rower, jogging outside), but you must keep a consistent pace, with your heart rate in the 120-to-130 range for at least 20 minutes.

WEDNESDAY: DELTOIDS AND BICEPS

Workout 1 (Preferably First Thing in the Morning on an Empty Stomach)

- 45 to 60 minutes of low- to medium-intensity cardio. Can be any variant that you like (stairs, treadmill, rower, jogging outside), but you must keep a consistent pace, with your heart rate in the 120-to-130 range for at least 20 minutes.

Workout 2 (Some Other Time During the Day)

- Dynamic Warm-Up

- Do an Ab Program. (See page 124.)

- Do the same workout from week 5, except cut down the rest time to 50 seconds.

- After the workout: Go directly into low- to medium-intensity cardio. Can be any variant that you like (stairs, treadmill, rower, jogging outside), but you must keep a consistent pace, with your heart rate in the 120-to-130 range for at least 20 minutes.

THURSDAY: CHEST AND BACK

Workout 1 (Preferably First Thing in the Morning on an Empty Stomach)

- 45 to 60 minutes of low- to medium-intensity cardio. Can be any variant that you like (stairs, treadmill, rower, jogging outside), but you must keep a consistent pace, with your heart rate in the 120-to-130 range for at least 20 minutes.

Workout 2 (Some Other Time During the Day)

- Dynamic Warm-Up

- Do the same workout from week 5, except cut down the rest time to 50 seconds.

- After the workout: Go directly into low- to medium-intensity cardio. Can be any variant that you like (stairs, treadmill, rower, jogging outside), but you must keep a consistent pace, with your heart rate in the 120-to-130 range for at least 20 minutes.

FRIDAY: LEGS AND TRICEPS

Workout 1 (Preferably First Thing in the Morning on an Empty Stomach)

- 45 to 60 minutes of low- to medium-intensity cardio. Can be any variant that you like (stairs, treadmill, rower, jogging outside), but you must keep a consistent pace, with your heart rate in the 120-to-130 range for at least 20 minutes.

Workout 2 (Some Other Time During the Day)

- Dynamic Warm-Up

- Do an Ab Program. (See page 124.)

- Do the same workout from week 5, except cut down the rest time to 50 seconds.

- After the workout: Go directly into low- to medium-intensity cardio. Can be any variant that you like (stairs, treadmill, rower, jogging outside), but you must keep a consistent pace, with your heart rate in the 120-to-130 range for at least 20 minutes.

SATURDAY: DELTOIDS AND BICEPS

Workout 1 (Preferably First Thing in the Morning on an Empty Stomach)

- 45 to 60 minutes of low- to medium-intensity cardio. Can be any variant that you like (stairs, treadmill, rower, jogging outside), but you must keep a consistent pace, with your heart rate in the 120-to-130 range for at least 20 minutes.

Workout 2 (Some Other Time During the Day)

- Dynamic Warm-Up

- Do the same workout from week 5, except cut down the rest time to 50 seconds.

- After the workout: Go directly into low- to medium-intensity cardio. Can be any variant that you like (stairs, treadmill, rower, jog outside), but you must keep a consistent pace, with your heart rate in the 120-to-130 range for at least 20 minutes.

SUNDAY: EXTRA CREDIT

Workout 1 (Preferably First Thing in the Morning on an Empty Stomach)

- 45 to 60 minutes of low- to medium-intensity cardio. Can be any variant that you like (stairs, treadmill, rower, jogging outside), but you must keep a consistent pace, with your heart rate in the 120-to-130 range for at least 20 minutes.

- Do an Ab Program. (See page 124.)

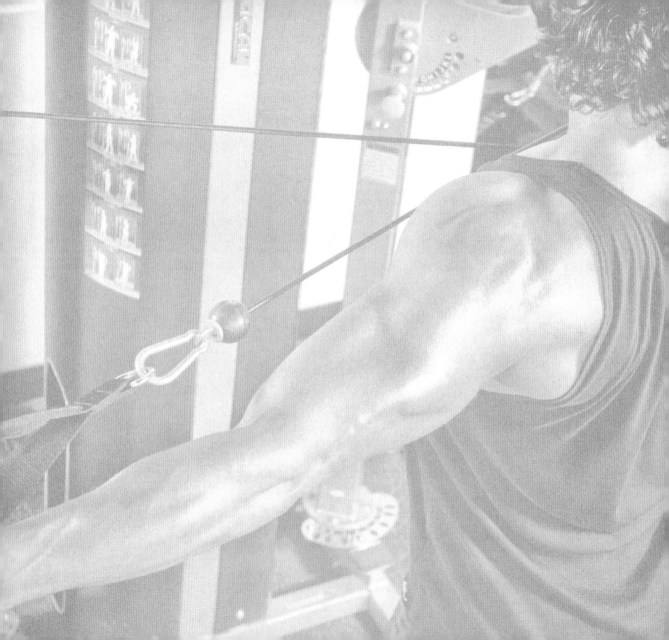

CHAPTER 7

Evolve
Your Eating

ut of all the areas of fitness that have required a lot of work, diet has thankfully been the easiest for me. In that respect, I know I'm the exception to the rule.

For most people, diet is the *biggest* hurdle and the most common reason why they don't look the way they want. That's because it's common for people to underestimate how much diet really controls the way you look. And how even by eating healthy, you're not necessarily taking in the types of foods—or the right amount of food—needed to maximize your training and look a particular way. There are plenty of healthy foods that won't push you closer to the image you want to see in the mirror.

Growing up, I was incredibly fortunate to have the mother that I did. I never ate poorly. She cooked every meal for my brother and me, using organic foods almost exclusively. As a result, I don't really have what would be considered a sweet tooth. The famous story my mom likes to tell is how after a doctor's office checkup when I must have been three or four years old, they handed me a lollipop on the way out, and I held it up to her in confusion—I didn't know what candy was. Her conditioning made it easier for me to avoid sugars now, which is apparently a big problem for most.

Most people live on a diet of processed crap and sugar, leaving a desire for the foods that are the absolute worst for your body. What's more, we have a food industry that is so deceptive with its marketing that oftentimes it's almost impossible to tell whether something is good or bad for you.

That is why the best way to approach your diet is to *keep it simple*. Learning good eating habits is really no different from learning anything else in life. If too much is thrown at you, it can be difficult to make the right choices and eat what you need. Just think about math. Do you go straight from simple addition to calculus? Of course not. And yet, how often is addition all you need to get by and be a functioning adult?

It's the same with diet. There are levels of complexity that we could go into here, but I want to revolutionize the game by making this aspect incredibly simple. Sticking to the basics, I've found, will get you much further than confusing you with complex systems and extreme details.

Just as I drew a line in the sand with fitness information, I'm asking you to buy in completely to my approach to diet. That's not to say this is the only way to eat or be healthy; that was never in question. I'm telling you what worked for me. This is a proven way to get the type of results you want. You bought this book for a reason. So get ready to let go of your emotional attachment to food and start looking at it in a whole new light.

WHERE DID WE GO WRONG?

Just as the issues in the gym start with a lack of education, the same can be said about diet. Quite simply, people don't read food labels, and then they wonder why they get fat. If you want the easiest way to clean up your diet, read the labels. All the information is there! Once you know what to look for, you have no excuse for making the wrong decisions. Even if you don't understand the difference between protein, carbohydrates, and fats, look at the number of ingredients on the label. *Truth*: the more words and ingredients you don't recognize, the more likely it is that you're buying something you don't want to put into your body.

The biggest diet mistakes start and end with sugar. People eat way too much of it, and they don't realize how much of it is lurking in everything we consume. You can eat a "perfect" diet and pack your meals with proteins, healthy fats, and vegetables, but if you load up on sugar, it will undo everything. It's solely up to you to avoid sugar as much as possible. If you see it on food labels, avoid them or go for items that have the lowest counts—definitely less than 10 grams per serving. I prefer 0. The one exception will be fruits, which are sugary, but are allowed for 2 to 3 servings per day. Alcohol is a destroyer. Usually consumed at night and loaded with empty calories (and often sugary mixers), it turns to fat almost instantly and can undermine all of the training you are killing your-self over during the day.

Other mistakes you're likely to make are by-products of clever marketing. For instance, protein bars are some of the worst foods on the market. You just read that correctly: most protein bars are *bad*. They might be portrayed as a "health food," but the ingredient list of 95 percent of them would blow your mind. Oftentimes you'd be better off eating a Snickers candy bar.

The same can be said for protein shakes that are sold at health shops. There's nothing wrong with protein shakes; they're healthy, provide a good source of protein, and are convenient. But it's the execution—especially at most smoothie chains. Everything is fine when you start with a simple base of protein mixed in with water and maybe some real fruit. From there, things go wrong. Next thing you know, these smoothie shops have added three different syrups, three massive scoops of peanut butter, and some yogurt. And boom! Your small snack is now more than 2,000 calories and packs upward of 100 grams of sugar. So if you want a smoothie, just make it at home. It's much healthier, and it really doesn't take much time or effort.

In the end, once you've been armed with a little bit of information, the biggest mistakes you'll make are acts of laziness. Once you know to avoid sugar, it becomes easier to guide yourself toward the right options. A lot of people will complain that it's too expensive to eat healthy. While it can cost more, frozen options and bulk purchases for fruits, vegetables, and proteins—which you can find by shopping at Costco or Sam's Club—make it easier than ever for anyone to afford healthy foods. It's all about changing your routine. Once you do, you'll see how easy it can be.

If you're still concerned, don't be. As you're about to find out, I'll provide steps and rules that will make it realistic for you to know exactly what to eat, when to eat it, and how to make dieting frustration a thing of the past.

FEED THE ENGINE

I eat to build.

Four words that I've used repeatedly over the last five years. It's a mind-set that will help you understand food, take the emotion out of what you eat, and put intent into everything you consume. If something isn't going to add to my building process, then it's superfluous. There's no need to eat it, unless I'm making a special exception to ease up on my diet or taking one of my well-deserved cheat meals.

Remember, your diet is essential because it not only controls your aesthetics but also plays a big role in your overall health. Food controls many of your basic needs and drives. So when it comes to eating, the bigger question becomes, What do I want my quality of life to be?

Before we get into the specifics of the diet, understand the difference between eating a good diet and following an unrealistic plan. If I want dessert, I'll have a dessert. Or if I want bread, I'll have it. This plan is not meant to be unrealistic or overbearing. At the same time, it is a commitment. Desserts are not something that happens every day—far from it. Building a plan that works is about putting yourself in control over what you eat and put into your body, and not making the plan so inflexible that you go insane.

This plan is about mental toughness, but it's also about enjoyment and understanding the direct benefit of how much you'll get out of what you put into your mouth. It's basic ROI—return on investment—and it's something you can control directly.

The idea of control, or, rather, lack thereof, is essential here. Just think about it: there's probably 85 percent to 90 percent of life that is completely out of your control. You're not flying the plane in the sky. You're not controlling the crazy people in life, the horrendous drivers, and so on. These things are all beyond your power and a potential danger.

Your diet is also a potential danger. But you are in control of it. You can eat crappy food that is composed of completely empty calories, or you can eat stuff that helps you build your body. Which direction do you want to go?

DON'T PAY THE MINIMUM

You want to know why your diet sucks? You guessed it: mind-set. Most people are treading water, trying to make their bad decisions work for them. Lots of people eat for comfort, because it's a seemingly less damaging vice than some of the others they could be engaging in.

But you need to decide: What's more important—that McGriddle sandwich and hash browns or your perception of your life? If you want to change who you are and what you can achieve, how valuable is that McGriddle? If you have an opportunity to change how people view you and how you see and feel about yourself, how important are those extra snacks? For me, I'd rather skip dessert and allow my life to be something bigger. Because in the end, nothing is worth more than that.

Oftentimes we rationalize postponing long-term goals for short-term satisfaction. In reality, making sacrifices in the short term will result in long-term happiness. That's a trade I suggest you make every time. Trust me, it's worth it.

You are in a gym only one hour a day, and what you do with those other twenty-three hours are extremely important. This is the best way to understand why your diet matters so much. It's the bigger piece of the pie.

I think of training in terms of construction. When I work out, I'm building a house, and the food I eat is the raw material: the bricks that insure the house is built solid. Eating is a job. I know I'll work hard enough in the gym, but if I don't supply the bricks, it will take longer to build the house—or even worse, it may never be built at all.

Before I had this mind-set, I used to see what I could get away with. It was no different than how many people treat their credit cards. They open a card, run up the balance, and then pay the monthly minimum to keep the creditors off their backs. The fact is, those people will always be in the negative doing only what it takes to break even.

The same approach applies to your body. In my early twenties, I was working out to pay off the debt on the caloric credit card that I was drinking at night. I'd eat something I shouldn't or drink a bunch of booze, and then get up late and try to offset the damage with exercise. It was the "Just keep paying the minimum" mentality, and it kept me spinning at zero.

I could undo in a weekend what it took weeks and months to build up. That's why I never looked the way I wanted. That's why it took so long to see results. These days, everything is different. I'm thirty-six, and I see results easier and a lot quicker than I did ten years ago, because I've gotten a lot better at taking care of myself during those other twenty-three hours of the day. This also smashed my self-limiting belief about age. Getting older doesn't mean that you have to slow down. It just means you have to play the margins even closer.

SIMPLIFY YOUR EATING PLAN

There's a misperception that because I'm in shape, it's easy to look the way I do. The general public usually holds one of these two assumptions:

- I can eat whatever I want because of great genetics.

- I starve myself and live a deprived life, and it sucks.

Both of these beliefs are false. My appearance, unfortunately, didn't just "happen," but my diet isn't something that I hate or that leaves me wishing I had a different life or a different career. The perception that you have to starve yourself and be "manorexic" is ridiculous. Your body needs fuel to build muscle and to live.

I eat a ton, and if I don't eat enough, people close to me start to notice. My diet and workout plan are designed to raise my metabolism to a sometimes frightening rate. I'm frequently asked by waiters if my order was just for me or for the entire table.

My point here is this: if you're fueling your body the right way, you're not deprived, you're not hungry, and you're not unhappy.

It's just a matter of knowing what to eat and how.

Follow these dieting steps to simplify the process and make it easier to take on a new style of eating that you'll enjoy.

STEP 1: TRACK YOUR MEALS

The very first assignment Ron gave to me when we began training for *True Blood* was this, and now I'm giving it to you . . . "I want you to write down everything you eat for a week. If you eat cookies, write down cookies." And I mean everything! Specific and in detail. Just by tracking, you'll learn a lot about yourself, both in terms of what you eat and how willing you are to be honest.

I have an alarm that goes off whenever I'm cheating on my diet. It's a learned behavior from tracking, and one that allows me to decide if "cheating" is something I really want to do. That's why tracking is as much an exercise in awareness as it is in honesty and accountability. You'll become conscious of what you're eating and how much, and that will allow you to self-regulate and make changes. Most people will leave things off their list. Don't do that. It's like telling your doctor half of your symptoms. You're never going to get the correct diagnosis unless you're honest.

STEP 2: EAT ONLY WHAT YOU NEED

I learned the majority of my current eating strategy when I first started working with Dr. Mooney back in high school. He was the first person to teach me to eat frequently and strategically. Here was his plan: Dr. Mooney told me to cook massive amounts of chicken and veggies for the week and then portion out the foods by day into Ziploc bags and store them in the freezer. At the beginning of each day, I'd pull out a bag and take it with me.

Whenever I was hungry, I'd pull out the bag and eat some chicken breasts and veggies. Once I was satisfied, I'd put it away. When I was hungry again, I'd graze. This did two things: it taught me to eat frequently, but, more importantly, I was able to learn the point of satiety. You literally need to train yourself to eat to the point of satisfaction and then shut it down, in order to teach your body not to store anything extra. If it's constantly being fed small amounts all day, it won't need to keep extra stores. Most people eat until they're stuffed, and they don't understand how to recognize hunger. This is what leads to overeating and mistaken cravings.

Mooney's approach was perfect for me. It was good food that provided high-quality nutrition and plenty of "bricks" for muscle building. It's not exactly easy to become fat on a diet of chicken and veggies, coupled with vigorous exercise. At the end of the day, you'll feel amazing, healthy, and energized. Your body will be filled with protein, fiber, and micronutrients, which is exactly what you need to grow. Think of protein-rich food as newspaper thrown into a fire. It's fuel that burns fast. You have to constantly be ready to throw more in at a moment's notice, to refuel when needed.

That's not to say that you need to fill up bags with a week's worth of food like I did, but it gives you an idea of how far you can take it.

I'm also not saying that eating throughout the day is the only method that works. But after trying multiple diets and approaches, it's the one I found far and away the most effective and enjoyable.

Many people are aware of the strategy of eating frequent meals, but their execution is poor. Eat till the point of satiety, stop, and then resume eating when you are hungry again. This is not about eating as much as possible. Instead, listen to your body. If you prepared a certain amount of food and you're full before you finish, stop eating and save the food for later. Don't keep eating.

STEP 3: PROTEIN AND MORE PROTEIN

For the sake of keeping it simple, make sure that there's an abundance of protein in each meal you eat. Protein is a natural anabolic substance that helps you build muscle and burn fat. It helps keep you feeling full, too. I generally eat more protein at meals than my body can process completely, simply because it prevents me from filling up on other crap. When you're making dietary changes, you want to eliminate the extra calories that won't help you with your goals. Sugars have to go. So do bread, mayo, and alcohol. It all has to go. The problem is, if you're still hungry, it makes it easier for you to reach for these choices and ruin your progress. That's why protein is so important. If you're not hungry, you won't reach for extras. Plain and simple.

In general, I've always followed a pretty clean diet, but that's not to say I don't know what it's like to have cravings and not be satisfied. You're much less likely to rush to a fast-food joint and stuff your face when you're not hungry, and protein is one of the easiest ways to ward off that demon.

STEP 4: EAT VEGGIES AND FATS

Protein will be a staple of your diet, but the other elements of your diet that will allow you to transform are vegetables and fats. The vegetables should come as no surprise. In terms of understanding what you're eating, they will serve as your primary carb source and provide all the nutrition you need to stay healthy and lean while stuffing your body with protein.

Healthy fats are your secret weapons, because they are essential for testosterone production. I've never touched steroids, human growth hormone, or other performance-enhancing drugs, and yet I continue to grow bigger every year. How? Because I eat and train in a way that promotes natural hormone production. Healthy fats, like those found in grass-fed red meat and butter, olive oil, coconut oil, nuts, seeds, and avocados, promote the production of testosterone, especially when combined with strength training.

It's the reason why I eat foods like bacon and steak, why I cook my foods in olive oil and coconut oil, and why I constantly consume nuts such as almonds and Brazil nuts. This isn't a license to eat unlimited fat (which is why I eat egg whites if I'm having sausage, for example), but to eat healthy, moderate amounts.

Fats to avoid include all vegetable and soybean oils, as well as mayo and dressings made from them.

SAMPLE MEAL PLAN

Unlike many diet plans, I'm not going to have you count calories. Why? Because it's frustrating and boring, and you don't want to be that guy busting out the scale at a restaurant. Instead, I suggest you follow these rules and use my diet template to model your needs. Remember, this is about learning to listen to your body. In general, the approach is to eat three big meals and then fill the gaps with protein snacks.

Meal 1: protein bar (no sugar added)

Morning workout

Meal 2 (postworkout): protein shake

Meal 3 (1 hour after postworkout shake): egg whites-ham-and-cheese omelet with side of bacon or sausage, side of sautéed vegetables, and a cup of coffee

Meal 4: chicken breast and vegetables

Meal 5: steak and vegetables

Meal 6 (prebed): protein shake

CAN I CHEAT?

As I've mentioned before, this type of diet is meant to be strict yet flexible. While that might seem contradictory, it actually makes perfect sense. In order to look lean and muscular, you have to follow a good diet. You have to be consistent, and you can't make excuses. But if a plan isn't flexible, odds are you won't be able to stay on it for the long run. And since consistency is the foundation of success, you need a plan that you can adjust. Not to mention, if you're on target every day for every meal, it makes it much easier to provide yourself with leeway to enjoy one meal every week without any restrictions.

There are many reasons for this, and a lot of it has to do with the mental aspects of following a diet like this. Sometimes you are going to feel like an alien when you eat. Oftentimes you'll find yourself eating the same foods over and over again. Fortunately, they'll be foods that you enjoy and will find to be very filling, but any diet program can become monotonous. So it's nice to feel like a normal human being every once in a while and eat the burger with the bun or just taste something different that you haven't had in a while.

What's more, these cheat meals will feel like a reward. When you put in the hard work, you'll deserve things that feel good and remind you of your dedication. As a general rule of thumb, I like the idea of a cheat meal where you set the day and the time in stone, such as saying that every Saturday night is your cheat night, but that's it. This is something that I learned from my trainer, Ron, who, by the way, is

EVOLVE *WHAT YOU EAT:*

JOE MANGANIELLO'S EVOLUTION SHOPPING LIST

Steak*

Boneless, skinless chicken breast

Pork tenderloin

Bacon

Ham

Shrimp

Egg whites

Eggs

Almonds

Pistachios

Cashews

PB2 Peanut Butter

Cheddar cheese block

Goat cheese

Isopure 40-gram whey-protein o sugar protein drinks

Spring mix

Mixed greens

Spinach

Carrots

Celery

Sun-dried tomatoes

Bell peppers in all colors

Cucumber

Green onions

Yams

Sweet potatoes

Strawberries

Blueberries

Apples

Think Thin protein bars, peanut butter flavor

Zero-sugar nutrition bars

Sugar-free Jell-O

Sugar-free pudding

Roasted green and yellow squash

Coffee

Cherry-and-fig balsamic dressing

Greek yogurt

Oatmeal

40-gram whey-protein bars, low-sugar version

Low-calorie, low-sugar ice cream (5 grams sugar per serving, or less)

Sugar-free yogurt

* Bonus tip: You want to eat the exact steaks that I enjoy in my home? Go to the website of Omaha Steaks (www.omahasteaks.com) and buy the triple-trimmed filet mignon. It'll be one of the best steaks you can have in your own home. They also have the best boneless chicken breasts I've ever had in my life. You will not find a better piece of chicken anywhere.

the strictest eater I've ever seen in my life. If you make it more flexible and variable—such as taking a cheat whenever you feel like it—then you open the floodgates for more consistent cheating, which is exactly what you want to avoid. I suggest taking the emotion out of your eating. By providing that discipline, you won't slip up, and you'll enjoy the cheat meals even more.

Better yet? By maintaining a schedule like this, you'll find that you won't have the same urges or cravings. When you tell your body that cheat meals can happen at any time, you prime your body to desire the bad foods at any given moment. But when you build in structure, your body comes to know when it can go wild, much like a trained dog knows when to expect its food. This psychological process makes it easier on your body and can actually help kill cravings until your cheat day arrives.

THE ULTIMATE CHEAT MEAL

As for the meal itself, when I'm on a cheat, it's like *Man Versus Food*. Ideally, I'll head to Roscoe's House of Chicken and Waffles, a soul-food restaurant chain in California, and get the same thing each time. Here's how I like to reward myself. Because after all the work I put in, I deserve it.

MY ROSCOE'S CHEAT MEAL

Half a fried chicken

Two waffles with butter and syrup

Side of mac 'n cheese

Side of greens

Side of French fries

TRANSITIONING INTO THE EVOLUTION DIET

When I first started training with Ron, I learned some ways to fine-tune my diet, like cutting out rotisserie chicken and replacing it with a lower-fat oven-roasted style instead. It was tricky to give up some of the little things. That is, until I discovered a bunch of meal options that helped me wean myself off the foods I wanted but needed to ditch.

The first food was sugar-free Popsicles. If you struggle with sugar cravings, stock up on a few boxes. During my first year on *True Blood,* I was cutting down from what a trainer friend of mine, Johnathan, jokingly called a "bubbly" 240 pounds. In the beginning, I really wanted sugar, despite never really having been a guy who craved it. When I look back, it was mostly a mental block combined with all the hard training. But man, did I want something sweet! So I'd eat a sugar-free Popsicle at night or sugar-free Jello-O cups. They really helped satisfy my sugar desire, and eventually I no longer needed them at all.

Once you start adjusting to the new style of eating, do everything you can to make the diet easier to maintain. I keep foods around that are healthy and good for me. For instance, I keep bags of pistachios and raw almonds in my car. I drink a lot of Isopure protein drinks, which contain 40 grams of whey protein yet taste like Kool-Aid, with 0 grams of sugar. They are stocked in my house at all times.

I'm also a fan of the Weight Watchers peanut butter cups without sugar and Arctic Zero ice cream. These things might seem ridiculous, but it's what you might need to make the process easier. Stack the deck!

WHAT ABOUT SUPPLEMENTS?

I'm not a guy who takes many supplements, simply because I don't think there are many that are necessary or work, for that matter. A lot of the supplement industry is just marketing, and I don't want to take anything that doesn't have a lot of proven effectiveness. Here's what I take:

Creatine: it builds muscle and helps with recovery.
How much: I take 5 grams before my workout and 5 grams after. Sometimes I add another 5 grams before I go to sleep. Go-to brand: Kre-Alkalyn.

Whey protein: it helps build muscle and insure that you get enough protein in your diet.
How much: I take protein after my workouts and throughout the day as snacks between meals. Go-to brand: Isopure.

Glutamine: good for your immune system and recovery.
How much: I use about 10 grams after a workout and before I go to sleep.

Nitric oxide-releasing supplement: helps me with recovery and before a workout.
How much: 1 serving before a workout and then later on in the day. Go-to brand: Nitrix.

Caffeine: some might not consider it a supplement, but you might as well toss it in here. It's probably the best performance enhancer science has found.
How much: a few cups of coffee before weight training or cardio.

THE DIET RULES SIMPLIFIED

This section is for anyone who still thinks there's some magic behind what I eat. If you follow these quick-start rules, it will be nearly impossible for you to screw up your diet.

Rule 1:   Always have three big meals per day.

Rule 2:   Fill your hunger gaps with small snacks that include protein.

Rule 3:   Protein, protein, and more protein at all meals.

Rule 4:   Kiss sugar good-bye.

Rule 5:   Drop the alcohol.

Rule 6:   Eat fiber from various sources (nuts, fruit, vegetables, berries, legumes)

Rule 7:   Vegetables at every meal.

Rule 8:   Don't avoid foods that include saturated fat such as fish, beef, pork, and eggs.

Rule 9:   Drink water throughout the day. If training, aim for 3 liters per day.

Rule 10: Limit carbs to natural sources such as sweet potatoes.

Rule 11: When not preparing for an event, enjoy one cheat meal per week.

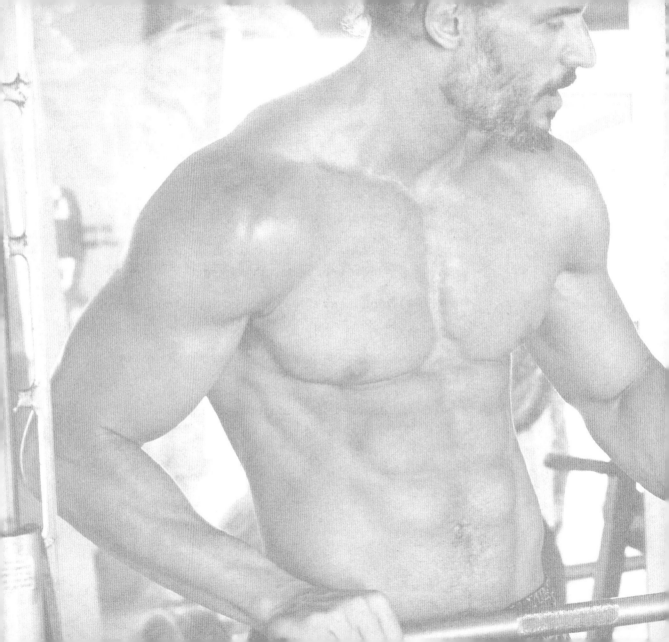

CHAPTER 8

Mission Possible: Getting Abs

There's a reason why so many guys have trouble seeing their abs, and it has nothing to do with the type of exercises they perform. Instead, it's that most guys are misinformed about what it takes to make their abs pop. Even with the best workout program and exercises that will make your core scream, it's the diet and cardio that are needed for you to see the muscles in your midsection.

When I first started on *True Blood,* I had put on some empty weight and was pushing the scales at a not-very-defined 240. Knowing the nature of the show and the role I was playing, I knew right away that I was going to be naked—a lot. Up until that point, I had been lifting for size, and my abs were nowhere near where I wanted them to be. The strange truth was that being big and muscular was now the easy part for me. Maintaining that size *and* at the same time having ripped abs was going to take some planning and discipline. My ab training would consist of training them efficiently, activating the muscles in my abdomen at full capacity, and, most importantly, burning away all the layers of fat that were covering the deep cuts of the muscles, so that the camera could see them.

At the end of the day, you can have the strongest abs in the world, but if you have too much fat on your body, you won't see them. Power lifters are the perfect example. At first glance, those guys look muscular but kind of fat. From a strength standpoint, they have insanely strong, powerful, dense abs for hoisting and holding those incredibly heavy weights. The big difference is that their diets aren't designed to strip fat, and their cardio (if they do any) isn't designed to cut them up. The point being, if you want to see your abs, those elements are necessary to bring them to the surface.

AB TRAINING 101

Your abs are a very complex grouping. There are several layers, cross sections, and muscles that combine to make them up.

Former NFL football star running back Herschel Walker, now a mixed martial artist, was famous for doing a thousand sit-ups per night. It was his accomplishment on the gridiron that gave the perception that doing an insane number of daily abs excercises was the only way to go. And while Herschel is a physical specimen, you don't need to do a Herschel-type workout to blast your abs.

I don't do a Herschel Walker amount of abdominal crunches. I work my abs three times per week, but I hit them hard and efficiently. I used to do abs after my workout, but I think it's smarter to do them before, because any workout worth anything is going to engage your abs—especially the workouts in this book. For example, even when you're doing biceps curls, your abs are engaged. So if you wear them out first, they're really going to have to work as they try to keep your core stabilized during your workouts.

Here's a huge trick to developing abs. Think of them as being like the reverse of a lobster's shell or your own vertebrae. If you imagine that your head is heavy like a bowling ball and lower it down from the top of where the first vertebrae meets the skull, and then lowering it farther and farther until it is down around your waist, you will start to feel the abs engage. This is the way to visualize them while working the basic crunch movement.

JOE MANGANIELLO'S FAVORITE AB ROUTINES

ROUTINE #1

A) Hanging Leg Raises (15 reps)

B) Hip-ups (20 reps)

C) Bicycles (25 reps)

D) Crunches (30 reps)

Perform all four of the exercises as a circuit, with no rest in between. Rest for a minute and then repeat two more times for a total of three circuits.

ROUTINE #2

A) Toes to Bar (15 reps)

B) Reverse Bicycles (25 reps)

C) Mountain Climbers (20 reps each side)

D) Crunches (30 reps)

Perform all four of the exercises as a circuit, with no rest in between. Rest for a minute and then repeat two more times for a total of three circuits.

With any abs movement, I imagine the top abs crunching into the middle, to the lower, to the start of the eight-pack. By that rationale, if you're targeting the lowest ab that crunches into the eight-pack, you're going to get them all and work your entire core region. That focus will make you work harder, cause your muscles to contract more forcefully, and produce changes that you will have to see to believe—and see them you will.

THE ROAD TO ABS: CARDIO

If you're serious about seeing your abs, do *not* skip this section. I don't care how much you hate cardio or think that weights and diet alone will do the job. They won't.

The intense program in this book will help you become lean, strong, and muscular. It will also improve your cardiovascular system by working at a fast pace with little rest, but this isn't your traditional lifting approach, where you sit around with your buddies and talk for three minutes between sets. The pace is quick, and the exercises—such as the heavy lifts—will tax your abs in ways you've never felt before.

Yet even with all of that, there is still a need for cardio. Does anyone like cardio, other than runners? I haven't met many. And according to my brother, who was a Division 1 middle-distance runner at Penn State University, even runners don't like it that much. For a long time, I compared treadmills to being a caged hamster on a wheel. It was boring, painful, and didn't seem like it did any good, but I have learned to make it work for me, and I've accepted it as a necessary part of my own Evolution.

The toughest aspect of cardio is getting moving in the beginning. Sir Isaac Newton's First Law of Motion states that an object at rest will stay at rest unless an external force acts upon it. In other words, it's hardest to get something started, but once you do and it's up and moving, it is infinitely easier to keep it going.

Like any form of exercise, if you do cardio consistently enough, your body starts needing it, wanting it, and getting excited to do it. Remember my morning construction headaches? Trust me, your body will acclimate, but it might take some time.

ALL IN

You might be telling yourself that you don't need to be on-screen and go that extra mile, and therefore you don't "need" cardio. That might well be true, but then this entire time reading would have been a waste. I am of the same school of thought as Dr. Mooney and Ron. They didn't pull punches with me, and I'm not going to with you. Dr. Mooney told me that I would see results only if I went all in, and years later, Ron told me the exact same thing, and I followed their directions to a T. I'm now demanding the same of you. You've got the information, you know better. *All in*.

It's best in this case if you think less and do more. I try to keep my brain out of it, in terms of training. Because if I think about it, odds are I'll *overthink* it. Keep it simple. I committed to a workout program, and there's a reason why they call it a workout *program*. It's not a workout feeling or whim.

Cardio sucks at the beginning, but what can you do? Accept that it's part of the process. This is truly where the men are separated from the boys. Cardio is the one thing you try to avoid the most, and it's quite possibly the biggest part of what you need for muscle separation and that ripped-abs look. Cardio is what will help you stand out from the pack.

Why go this far and not do it all the way? Why run a twenty-six-mile marathon and then say, "Screw the last two-tenths of a mile"? Make the investment. You either want it or you don't. If you want "Holy shit!" results, then this is not optional. It's a requirement that you *owe to* yourself. See what can happen. Release those mental blocks. Unshackle those fears. Stop talking about what you *could* be if you just did this or that. Finish it. Become it.

I'm telling you, it's been worth every grueling second. After my first season on *True Blood*, I netted $0 financially. Literally. After taxes, agent fees, manager fees, and life expenses, there was barely anything left. All I had, I invested in my trainer and an elliptical machine. I was putting that money right back into myself. I couldn't afford a Ferrari at the time, so I decided to build a Ferrari engine inside of me. I was gambling on the idea that if I built myself into the strongest, most badass version that I could on the inside, then that would ripple out and affect every aspect of my life. My life would have no choice but to match externally the improvements I was making internally. In his January 1993 *Details* magazine essay titled "The Iron," Henry Rollins wrote, "I believe that when the body is strong, the mind thinks strong thoughts . . . there is no better way to fight weakness than with strength. Once the mind and body have been awakened to their true potential, it's impossible to turn back." I put in every ounce of effort that I had—and it worked.

Make your body a priority. It doesn't need to be every last cent you own, but it should be important enough that you don't allow mental weakness and excuses to stand in the way.

True Blood was my pocket aces hand, and I put it all on the table. Are you willing to bet on yourself? If the answer is yes, don't skip the cardio. Make the commitment and eliminate your excuses.

ADDING CARDIO TO YOUR ROUTINE

Not doing cardio was one of the big barriers that separated me from my potential, and the way I saw it I had two choices: keep making excuses, or just suck it up and get it done. It was my own personal form of tough love that allowed me to remove the excuses and break through. Even then, I knew it would be difficult to force myself to do cardio, so I made an investment. I rented an apartment right across the street from an affordable gym—much to the chagrin of my then-girlfriend, who proceeded to complain about it every single day. With the immortal words of Don Swayze ringing in my ears, I eventually let that girl go, and thus freed up a ton of psychic energy. As a result, my career skyrocketed. Hey, you're either in the boat, or you're not. After that first season, *True Blood* offered me a six-year contract, including a signing bonus that I used to buy my very own elliptical machine. I could wake up and do morning cardio immediately, thus adding precious extra time to my day. And as an added bonus, I was also free to move wherever I wanted, because I no longer had to live across the street from a gym. Maybe you can't afford to buy a machine for your house, but you *can* invest in a gym membership for about the equivalent of one dollar a day and, like I did, even go so far as to move across the street from one. Hold yourself accountable for your cardio sessions. If you're expecting extra hours to magically appear in your day . . . they're not going to. Sometimes *you* have to make them appear. *No excuses.*

Once I had the machine, it was time to take another step in making cardio easier. I moved my television in front of my elliptical, turned on ESPN, and worked out during *Sports Center*. I allowed the television to take my mind *off* of the monotony of the cardio I despised doing and, once again, the beauty and satisfaction of earning the money to buy my own cardio equipment paid dividends in that I never again had to argue over switching off women's daytime programming to watch what I wanted to at the gym. The real miracle here was that eventually cardio became like a morning meditation. I really started enjoying it, and the results on my physique were astronomical. I began to look forward to getting up, getting a sweat in before breakfast, and then starting my day.

FAT-BLASTING CARDIO

I recommend adding cardio anywhere from three to six times per week. Just throw on your shoes and make it to the gym or find some space outdoors. I prefer indoor cardio, because modern technology allows you to manage every training variable, and it's easier to monitor growth. If you do this as I've prescribed below for one to two months, you will see a noticeable difference that you would not have otherwise. If you're overweight, you'll drop extra pounds. If you're healthy but not lean, you'll start to see more muscle. If you're lean, well, you're going to get absolutely shredded.

Go that extra mile and burn more calories. Here are three different ways I recommend to add cardio to your routine. Each has its benefits. Switch it up by mixing all three types into your program.

Cardio Option 1:
Elliptical: Early Morning Slow Cardio (45 Minutes)

This is *not* intense. Rather, it's a steady approach to getting your body moving first thing in the morning, preferably before you eat anything. I recommend moving at a pace that keeps your heart rate anywhere between 125–135 beats per minute and a resistance level of around 10. You'll hear a lot of people insult slow cardio, but I'm here to tell you it has a place at the table in the fat-burning process. Especially when your goal is abs and you want to leave nothing to chance.

Cardio Option 2:
Treadmill: High-Intensity Intervals (30 Minutes)

A warning: this is not for the faint of heart. Sprinting is one of the best ways to get in shape. This is a fast-paced, intense approach that will help scorch any unwanted fat from your body. When you perform this type of exercise, I want you to think of Olympic sprinters and their lean, chiseled bodies. No fat, all muscle. Those are bodies that are built with short-duration bursts of exercise performed at the highest intensity possible. You'll be left gasping for air, but your body will transform right in front of your eyes. If you are significantly over-weight, you might need to avoid this at first and build your foundation at a slower pace. Don't worry: everything is relative to your own body, which means that as long as you push as hard as your body allows, you will see results.

Here's how I approach interval sprints on a treadmill, but feel free to adjust to your own ability or do the same workout outdoors:

Warm-Up

- Set the treadmill at 7.5 miles per hour, with no incline.

- Jog for 5 minutes.

Interval Phase 1

- Set the treadmill at 10 miles per hour with a 7.5 percent incline.

- Run for 15 seconds and then step off for 45 seconds. That's one round. Complete ten rounds.

Interval Phase 2

- Set the treadmill at 12 miles per hour with a 10 percent incline.

- Sprint for 10 seconds and step off for 50 seconds. That's one round. Complete ten rounds.

Cooldown

- Set the treadmill at 7.5 miles per hour with no incline.

- Jog for 5 more minutes until your heart rate begins to lower.

Cardio Option 3:
Treadmill: High-Intensity Slow Cardio (30 to 45 Minutes)

This one can be deceptively nasty. I'll jump on the treadmill for a special type of fat burning. Here's how it works: I'll set the speed at 3.5 (brisk walk), pump the incline up to 12 percent, and set a timer for anywhere from 30 to 45 minutes. Think of this as walking uphill on a steep incline for a long period of time, like Rocky Balboa climbing the mountain in Russia in *Rocky IV*.

This might not seem like much, because during the first 5 minutes you feel fine. At right about 10 minutes, your body will hit its first wall. By 20 minutes, your body and your legs will be screaming. But if you can make it past the 20-minute barrier, you'll be amazed that you'll feel like you can go on forever. So keep pushing, remember your goal, and fight through until the timer goes off.

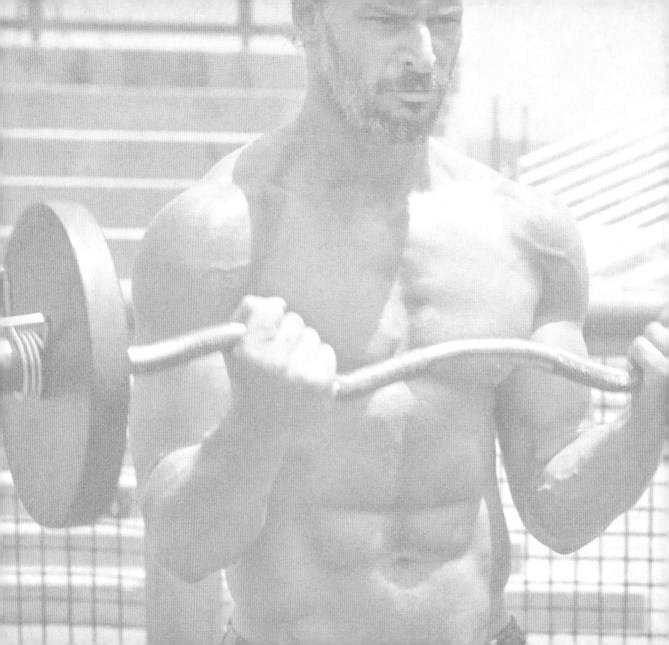

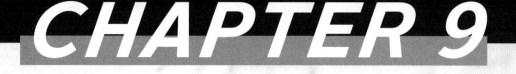

CHAPTER 9

Massive, Shredded, and Looking Your Best

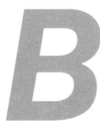

By this time, your mind is right, and you've started to look and feel great. I included this chapter as the absolute final frontier. This is the showroom-quality wax job. This chapter includes some tips and tricks utilized by bodybuilders and fitness professionals, with a little added modern flair. These are the finishing touches that will have people wrongly convinced that you got your physique through some unnatural way, like body makeup, airbrushing—even CGI.

PREPARING FOR A SHOOT

When I know that I have to be shirtless, everything gets kicked up another notch. There's no room for error. Everything, from my diet to my training, has to be perfect. "Film is forever," after all. In terms of my workouts, I institute "two a days," six days a week. Each day includes weight training *and* cardio.

This is the point where my workouts shift in their general nature. Because the camera picks up separation in your muscles, I focus less on increasing weight and raise the intensity by doing more reps and resting less. In other words, the philosophy is *constant motion*, a higher heart rate, and a big pump felt in every muscle.

At this stage of the game, I try to "circle the runway" of peak condition year-round. So if you're still on your way to your own personal peak, these strategies will help, but they won't have you razor sharp. Instead, use this approach once you have already gone through the 6-week program and are ready to put on that final coat of polish.

HIGH-DEFINITION PREPARATION ROUTINE

Wake-up	Take nitric oxide-releasing supplement and creatine.
Morning workout	Do cardio on the elliptical for 45 minutes (follow Cardio Option 1).
Breakfast	Egg-white omelet with cheese and green onion. Side of 2 sausages, a cup of sliced fruit, 50 grams of whey mixed with water, and black coffee.
3 hours later	2 oven-roasted chicken breasts with a side of corn and a side of steamed green beans.
Preworkout	Take nitric oxide-releasing supplement and creatine.
Workout	Weight training.
Postworkout drink	Lean Body.
2 hours later	1 Isopure RTD liquid protein drink and cut-up carrots, celery, peppers, and cucumber eaten with hummus.
2 hours later	Roasted pork loin with spinach, prosciutto, and goat cheese. Mixed green salad on the side with roasted squash.
Right before bed	Another 50 grams of whey protein mixed with water.

WHAT IF I TRAIN IN THE MORNING?

Oftentimes my day starts bright and early with a lifting workout with my trainer. In those situations, I'll have either the whey protein with water or a Lean Body and a Think Thin bar on the way to my workout. This will all be combined with the nitric oxide-releasing supplement and the creatine.

Then, once my training is complete, I'll start with breakfast and follow the rest of the day as shown. I'll also add my cardio during the afternoon where the weight workout is and follow that with the Lean Body, or I'll perform cardio right before dinner.

SHOOT DAY PREP

Everything in my diet is ultraclean leading up to a shoot. I *do not* eat any sugar, bread, mayo, or any sweets, treats, or carb sources besides berries and vegetables. This is done to prepare my body to look as good as possible during that moment the camera is on.

Cutting all carbs leading up to a shoot will do wonders for your body-fat percentage, but it can sometimes make your muscles look flat. Reintroducing sugar the day of the shoot can help to "superpump" your muscles while the sugar is in your system. This does cause an insulin surge—an important hormone that controls energy storage and reacts to carbohydrates—which can deflate you and bring about an energy crash, so for a long shoot, you have to be careful.

On the day of the shoot, I begin with a morning cardio session followed by a small breakfast of egg whites and a protein shake. After that, I don't eat until the shoot. I'll have plenty of time to stuff my face afterward, so discipline is key.

If you're doing a morning shoot, get up early, do some cardio, and then *don't* eat anything. You'll be enjoying some treats during the shoot to fill out your muscles, so just be mentally tough and ignore any hunger pangs.

During the shoot, I eat some sugar periodically: Jawbreakers and

Reese's Peanut Butter Cups are standard fare. The sugar will volumize your muscles when you're depleted and have amazing effects on a body that is lean and muscular and hasn't had carbs in a while. I'll also have some protein drinks on hand to sip on.

LOOKING YOUR BEST

Whenever I'm filming, I always bring a few pieces of equipment to insure that my muscles stay full of blood. I bring a BOSU ball (it's the ball that looks like half of a Swiss ball) and twenty-five-pound dumbbells with me to the set on the day of a shirtless shoot. Before shooting any given take, I crank out plyometric (bouncing) BOSU push-ups to the point of failure, then do regular (nonbouncing) push-ups on the BOSU to failure, to get as much blood as possible into my chest and triceps.

Then I perform some dumbbell push presses with the twenty-five-pounders, followed by front raises and lateral raises. This fills out my shoulders with extra detail and separation. The last piece of the upper-body blast includes some twisting curls, hammer curls, and curls with my arms twisted slightly out.

To finish off my preparation, I'll do a few crunches on the BOSU—but not many—and some triceps presses on a chair.

In terms of this approach, there's no need to take the pump to failure and do repetitions until you can't perform any more. So don't do as many reps as possible. Instead, do just enough reps to put some blood into your muscles and increase your vascularity. It's important to get a pump going and then use simple strategies to keep it so that you can look your best for a longer period of time.

To accomplish this goal, I stay pumped with some isometric movements, such as holding the weights in a contracted position (think the top portion of a curl). Or I'll press my hands together and squeeze every muscle in my upper body and arms.

WATER PILLS?

I'm not a water pill person. If you're thinking about cutting out water, be careful. Talk to your doctor. It can be extremely dangerous, and if done, should never incorporate water pills or any chemical diuretics. Also, make sure that the water cutting occurs about *twenty-four* hours out. After the shoot, you have to be very diligent about rehydration. Your body won't think twice about breaking down your hard-won muscle for the water and amino acids it desperately needs.

Prior to a shoot, I stop drinking any carbonation about a week out. And I also curb my water intake altogether about twenty-four hours out and use cardio to thin my skin out even further. I'm not completely crazy, though; I do sip water or protein drinks as needed on set, but very sparingly. The only "diuretic" I take are a few espresso shots on the day of the shoot.

WHAT ABOUT TANNING?

Tanning does help to bring out the definition and separation in your muscles. It creates shadows that enhance your overall physique.

And when I say tanning, I mean sun. Not spraytanned-on abs. If you're anything like me, you can spot fake abs and CGI definition a mile away.

AFTER THE SHOOT OR EVENT IS OVER . . .

This is when the fun begins. Reward yourself for your hard work! This is not falling off the wagon. It's a one-time splurge that you've earned before getting back on the program. After that much discipline, you deserve it! It's fried chicken 'n waffles time, baby!

GO BIG OR GO HOME

When it comes to the battlefield of gaining mass and becoming bigger, I am no stranger. Don't forget my humble beginnings as that skinny teenager. True, I've made huge strides since then, but my need to gain size isn't limited to my youth. When I was preparing for *Sabotage* with Arnold Schwarzenegger, I wanted the increased intimidation factor of being "linebacker big." I was playing a DEA agent who works undercover in a biker gang. For my physical training, I turned to powerlifting and Olympic lifts in the morning, then I would head over to the martial arts studio for ninety minutes of stand-up and ground-fighting MMA rounds. The result of this brutal change-up in my routine? By the time I showed up on set, I tipped the scales at 250 pounds! The biggest I'd ever been, while retaining serious definition in my abs. While building for mass using the Olympic and powerlifting techniques, in conjunction with the grappling and hand-to-hand sessions, I was free to add more calories. There were two ways to do this: make all of my meals bigger and/or simply add more meals to the day. Eating like this became like a part-time job for me, and I loved every second of it!

Here's my biggest mass-gaining tip: Take in more carbs. You can't grow muscle and become significantly bigger without carbs. Some of these carbs can be healthy sources such as sweet potatoes and rice. But also feel free to experiment with less healthy options. When I'm gaining, here's a sample breakfast:

4 eggs over easy

2 or 3 pancakes or waffles with butter

Side of sausage and/or bacon

Side of fruit

Pot of coffee

The pancakes might seem like an unhealthy choice, but if you're training hard and going at max intensity, these carbs will be essential to your growth. If you want to still show some definition through this phase, I suggest the heavy cardio of boxing or MMA to help your body stay centered through a phase of such radical physical transformation.

CHAPTER 10

Evolved

"But if the courses be departed from, the ends will change. Say it is thus with what you show me!"

—Ebenezer Scrooge to the Ghost of Christmas Yet to Come in Charles Dickens's *A Christmas Carol*, 1843

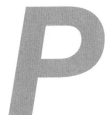eople can change. My life is living proof. I was young and stupid, and I got what young and stupid people get. But I found a way to change my perception, started operating from a different paradigm, opened a new chapter, and my life changed its course forever.

I wrote this book with the hope that my experiences and the lessons I learned along the way would inspire others to follow in my path . . . like a ghost of fitness yet to come, I'm here to hopefully guide you away from a possibly wasted future of doubt, regret, and *lost potential.*

You're at the point now where you know what needs to be done. Unlike before, you now have the solutions. You have been armed with all the information you need to create your own Evolution and step into the body and life you've always wanted. You'll be tougher, stronger, and more mentally prepared for everything that will come your way. You'll be ready to fail as a means to succeed, compete, rise to the top, and join the ranks of a new generation rocketing toward a more driven end. No more settling for less. No more being okay with something other than your best. No more stopping just because it gets tough, you have a bad day, or you think that the difficult road somehow won't be worth the effort.

It is.

It's time to evolve. Ask yourself: Do you want to keep getting the same results out of your workout and life? If not, are you willing to change it up? Are you willing to bring the intensity and focus to the gym as if your life depended on it? Are you willing to make the sacrifices at the altar of the dietary gods in order to once and for all get what's coming to you?

If you bought this book and have made it this far, then the answer is yes.

MAINTAINING YOUR FOCUS

Just because you've been given the knowledge to succeed, it doesn't guarantee success. Take it from me. I had that knowledge back with Dr. Mooney, but I let it slip away.

I transformed my entire body in preparation for my acting showcases upon graduation from CMU. The showcases, or Leagues, are where all of the graduating actors from drama schools from around the country perform for agents and casting directors in New York and L.A. It's like the National Football League Scouting Combine for young actors. You have three minutes onstage to make an impression. Three minutes to sum up four years of comprehensive classical theatre training in some of the greatest material ever written . . . unfortunately, none of which is appropriate to use in front of the agents and managers looking to fill out the casts of a host of contemporary projects. I had just spent four years being trained in classical material by some of the best acting teachers in the world, and no one in Los Angeles was going to give a shit about any of it. I considered what I could possibly show of myself in three fleeting minutes to give these people an idea of what I was capable of.

If the goal was to have every manager and agent want to sign me and every casting director want to call me in, I wanted it to be an absolute no-brainer . . . and then it hit me. If the goal was to get the attention from the crowd and separate myself from the herd in three short minutes, I wanted to do that as soon as I walked out on-stage. I wanted them to reach for their pens to check the box on their showcase forms to set up a meeting with me before I even opened my mouth, and then, once I did, have that seal the deal. I contacted the Moon Dog, and we got back to work. He got me dialed back in and in better shape than ever. Talent falls under the category of something that no one has any control over. It can be sharpened and refined by a training program like CMU's, but the only real variable under my control, as I saw it, and in terms of the showcases, was using my body to show my work ethic and marketability. I walked out onstage at the Leagues in a sleeveless shirt and then let my three minutes of work speak for itself. The response was exactly what I had hoped for. I wound up with my pick of agents and managers, as well as a slew of meetings with casting agents and directors. My professors at Carnegie Mellon said that it was one of the biggest responses in showcase history.

I was offered a TV deal that I turned down, because later that week, I was brought in to meet director Sam Raimi and screen-test for *Spider-Man*, in which he eventually cast me. I had it made—until I lost it all.

Once I reached some of my goals, I started hanging out with the wrong crowd and lost touch with that hungry kid who had fought so hard chasing his dream. I was staying out late, drinking a ton, and not sleeping enough. You know the quote, "Youth is wasted on the young"? That was me, and instead of becoming better and seeing what I could become, I spent too much time cleaning up the messes I was making. I knew the right path. I had seen it and lived it. But nonetheless, I proceeded to make my bed and then light it on fire.

I want you to avoid my mistakes. I'm living proof that the program contained in this book works. I'm an example of building myself up starting from the lowest rung possible, and then later in life falling even lower and having to do it all over again. I'm a living testament that once you get to the top, you have to keep going and keep fighting to grow, because the only way to coast . . . is down.

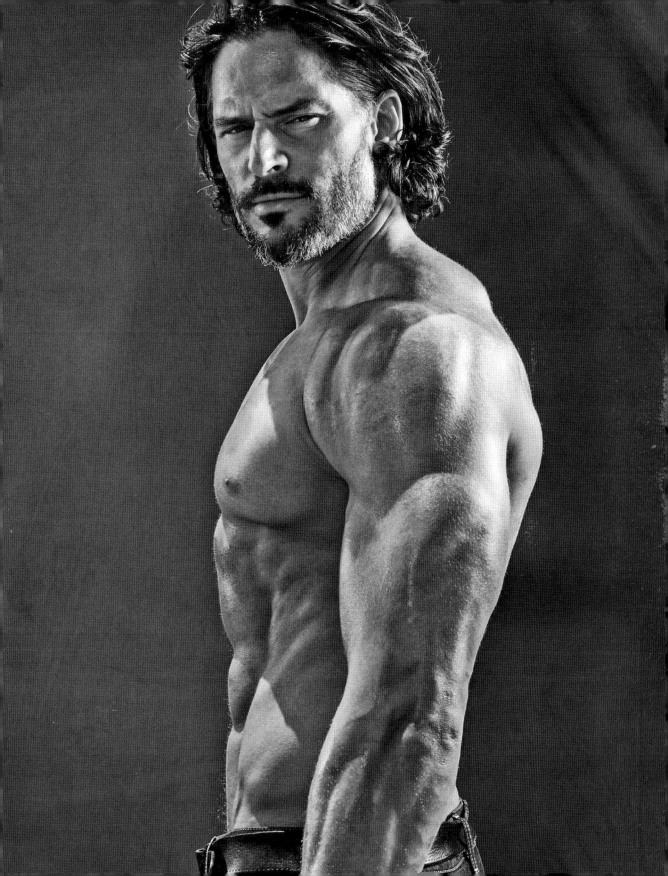

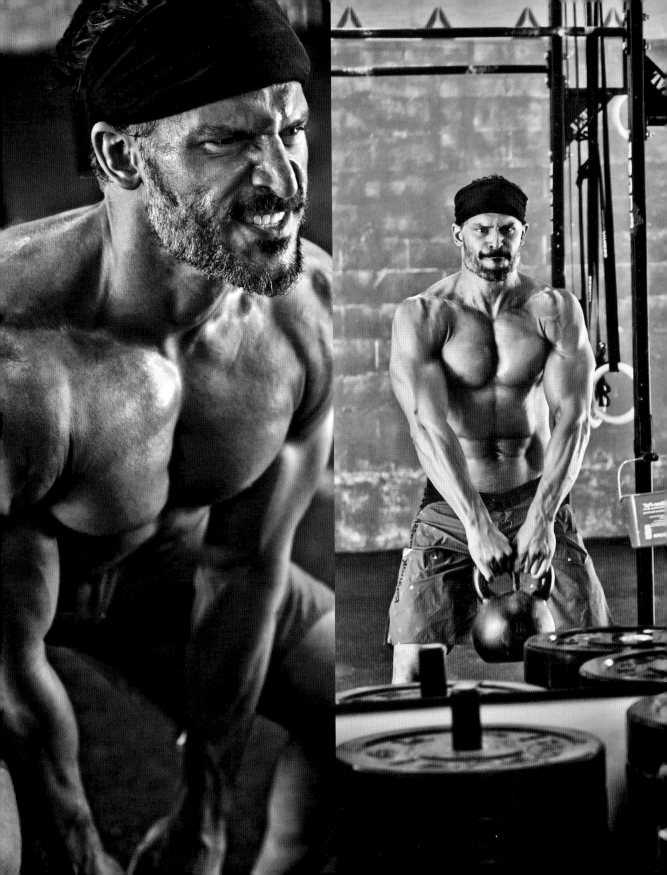

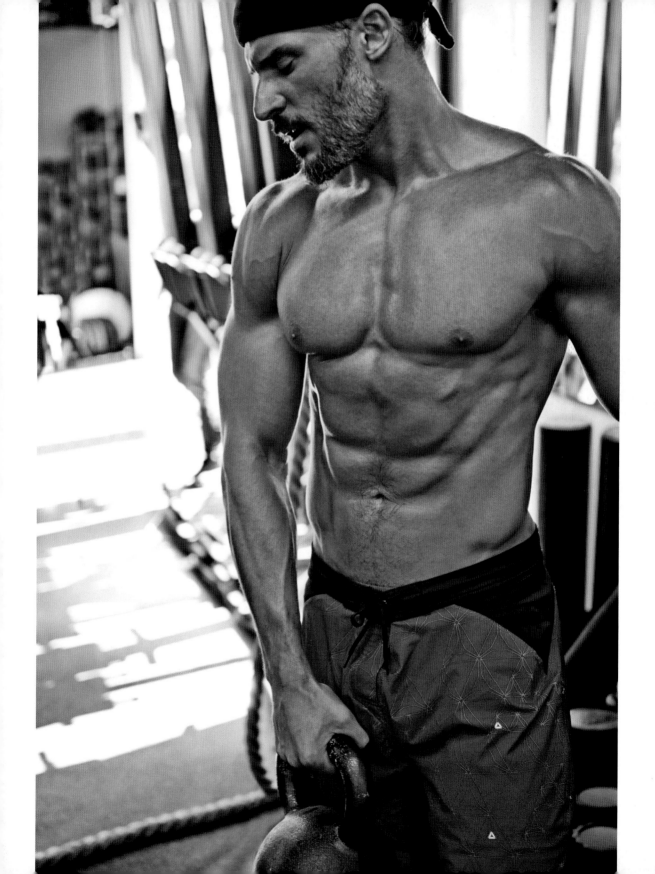

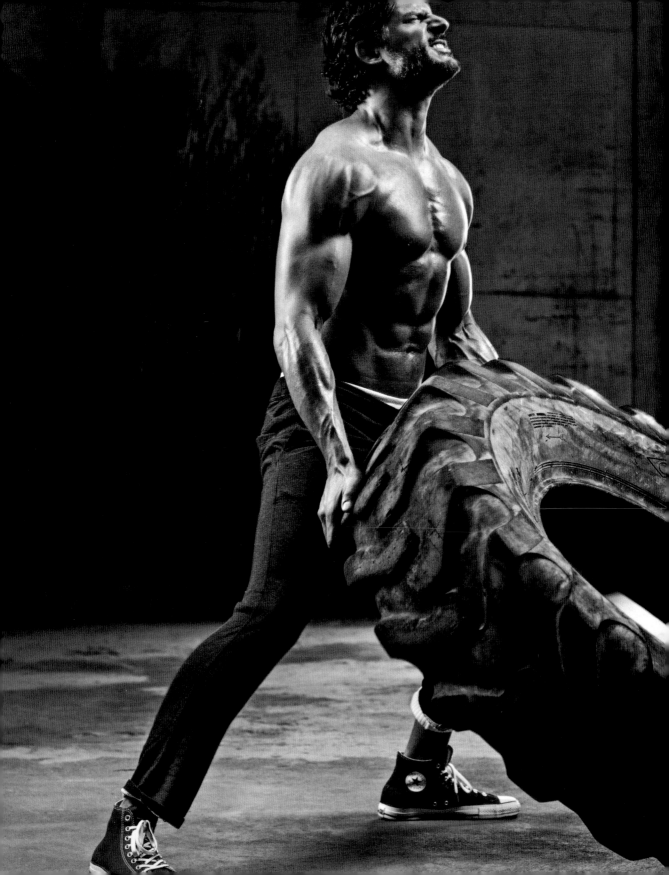

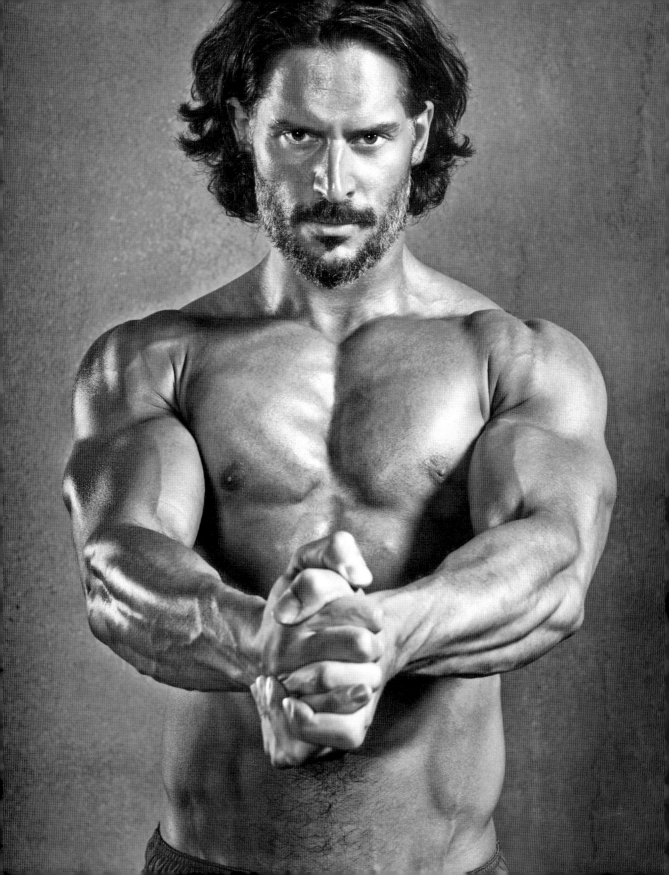

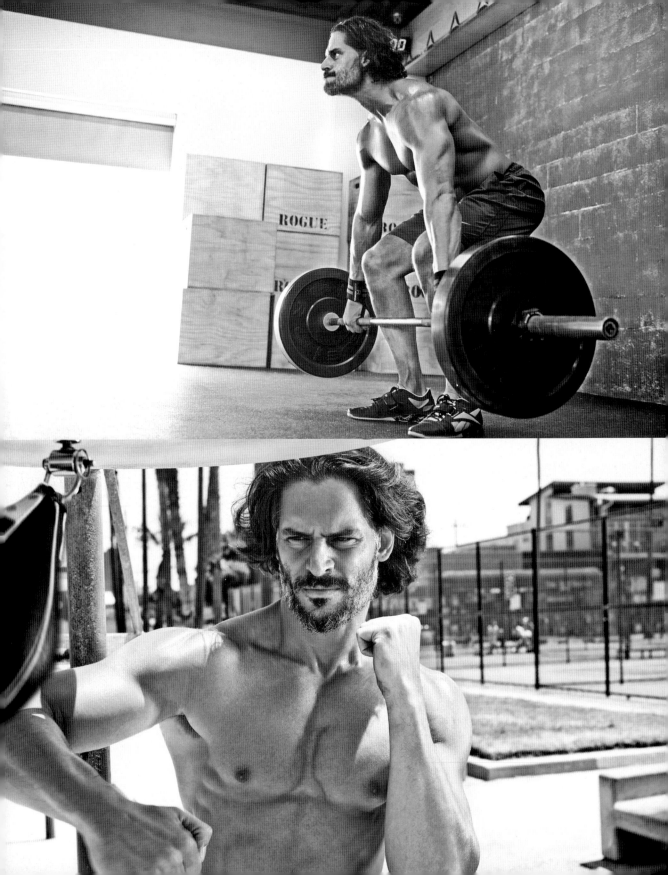

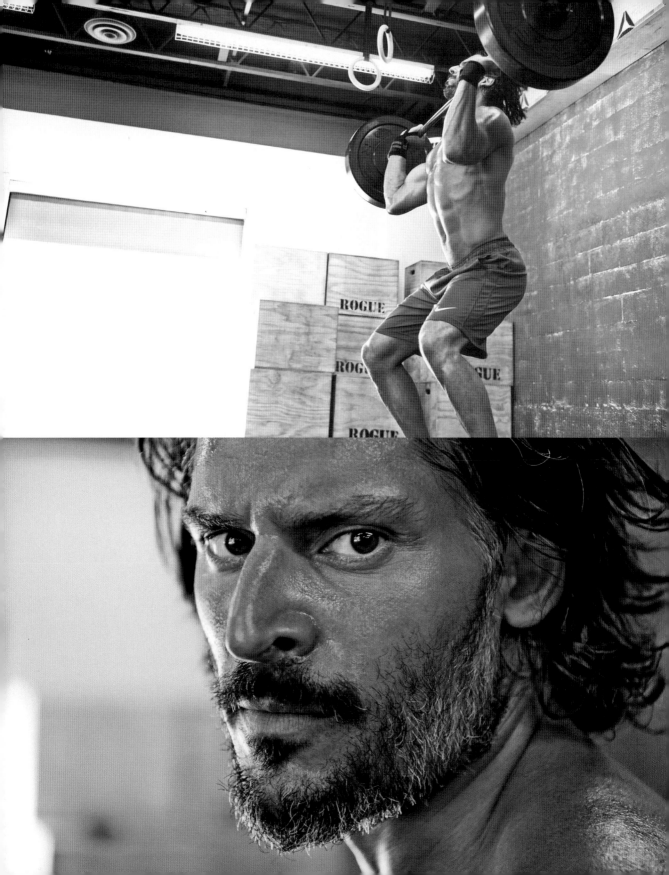

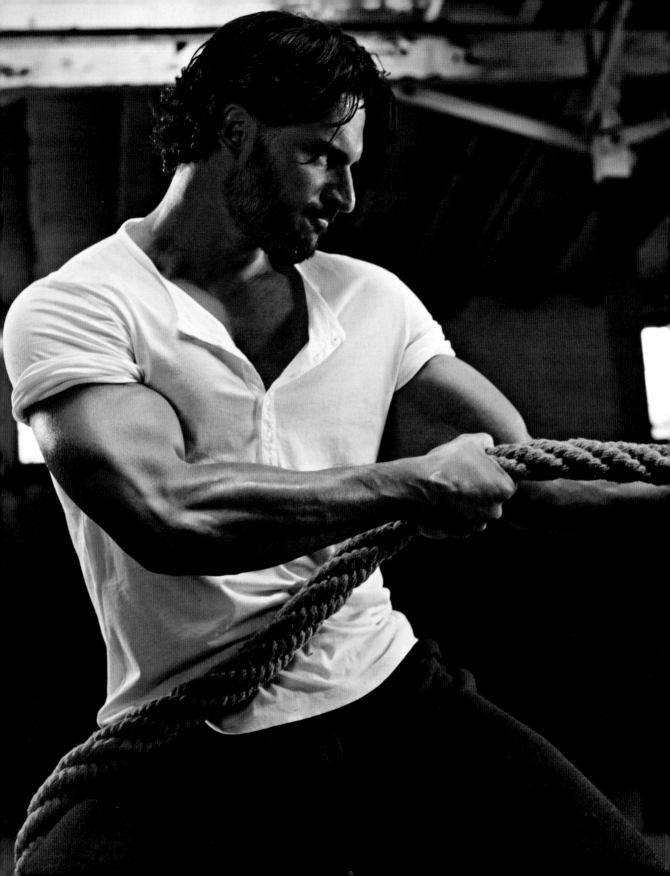

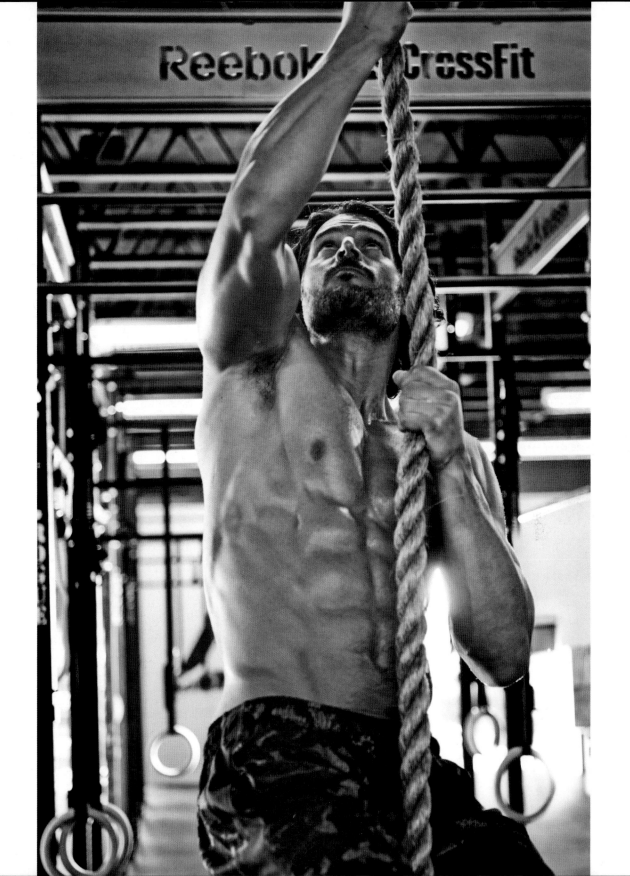

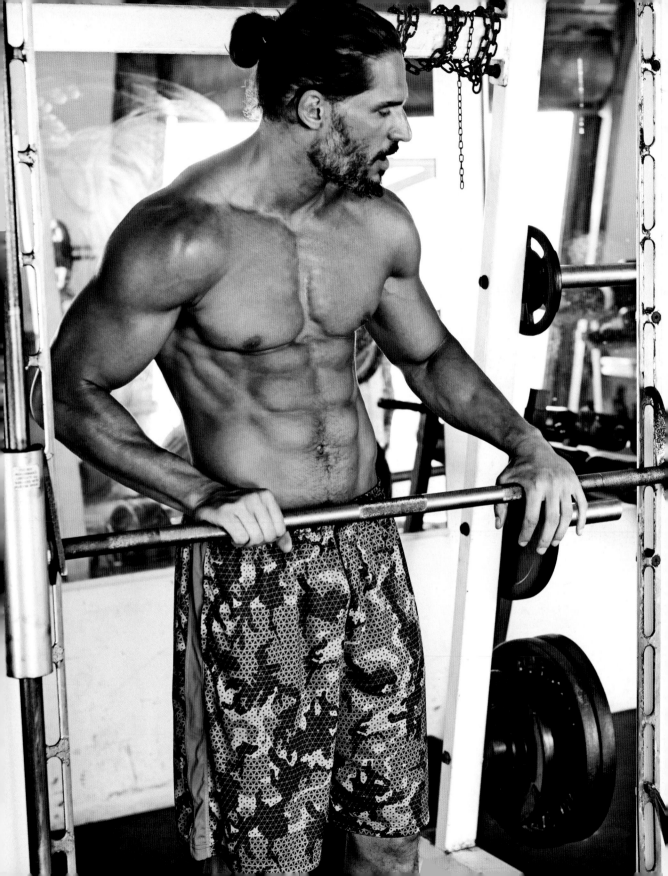

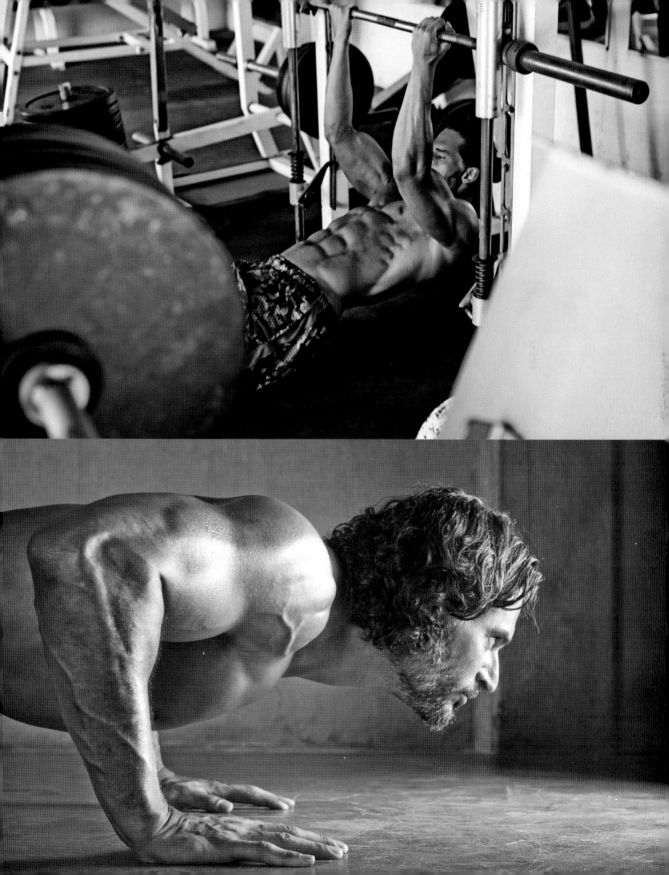

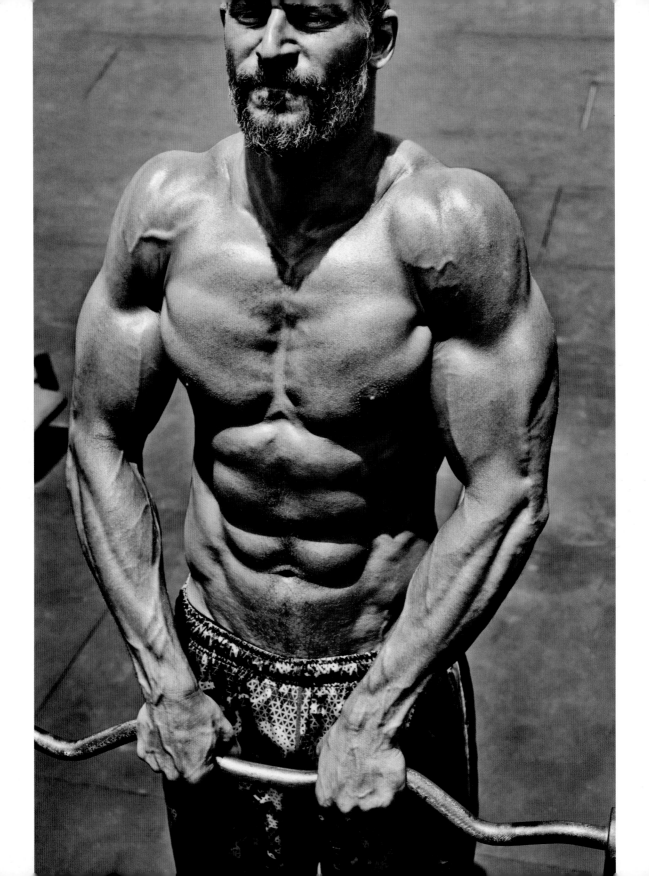

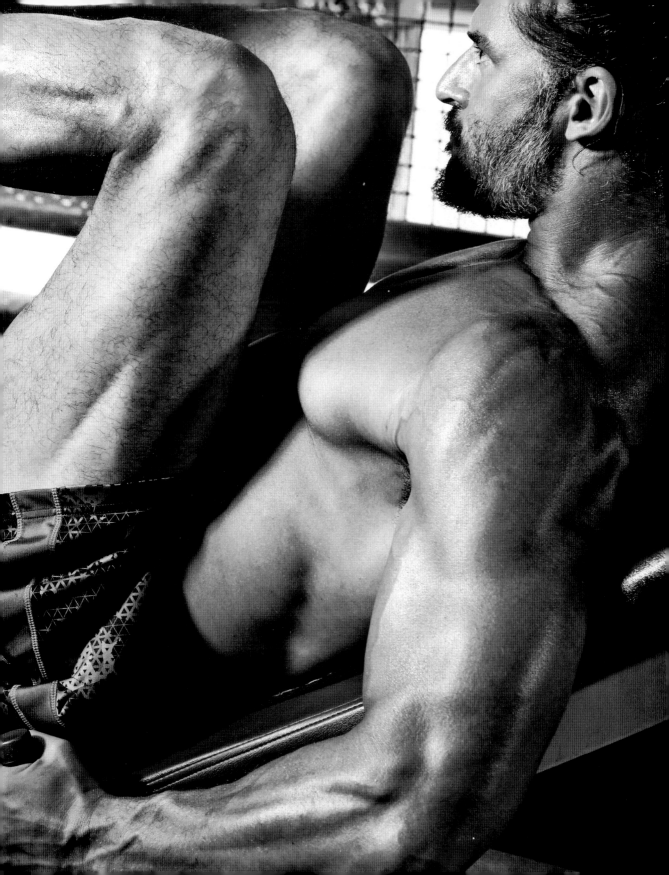

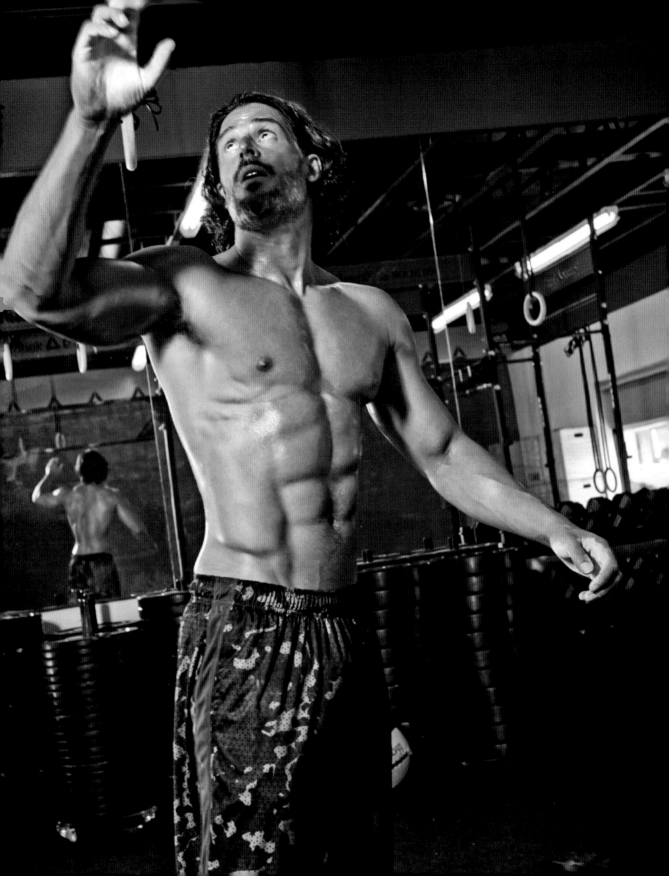

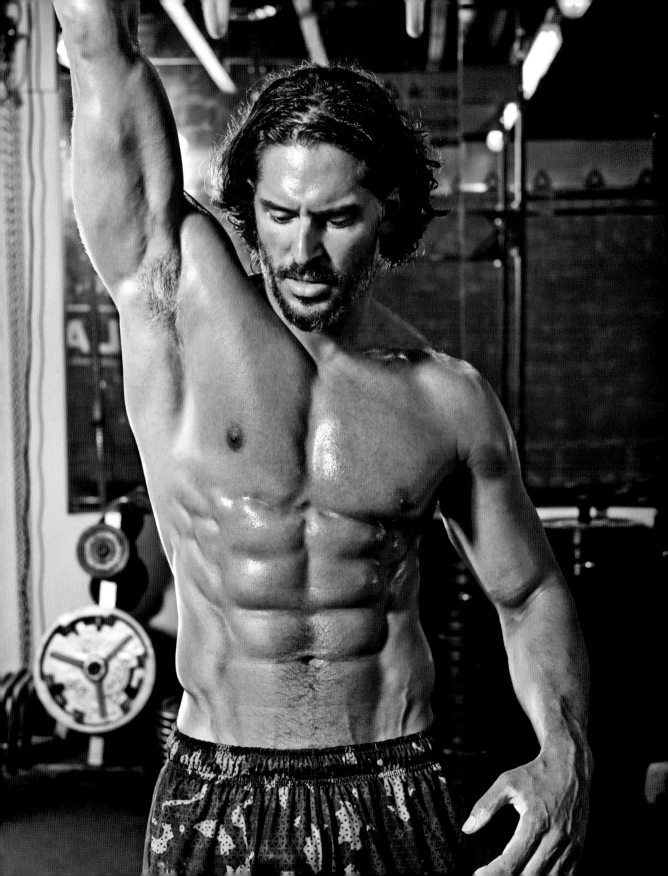

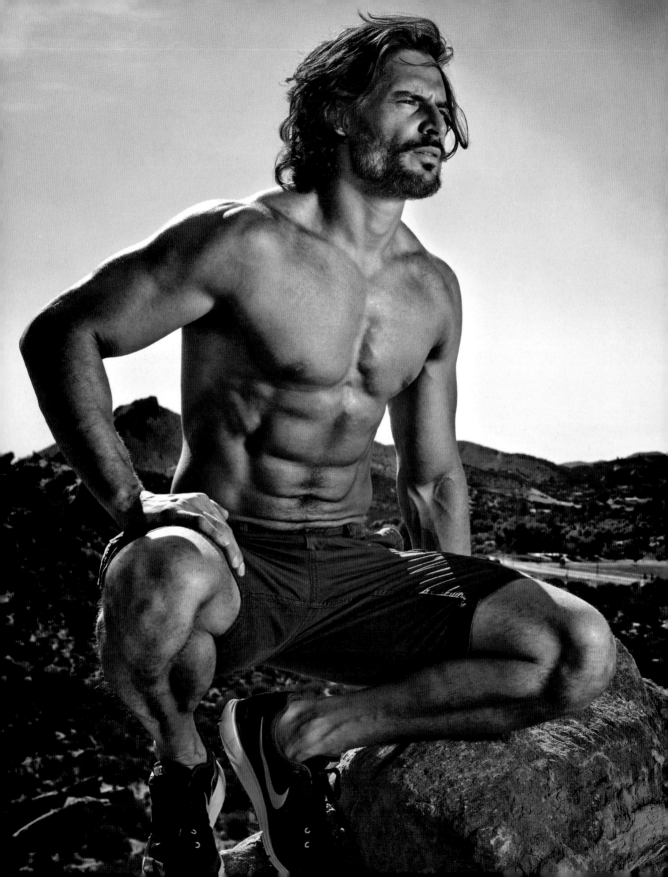

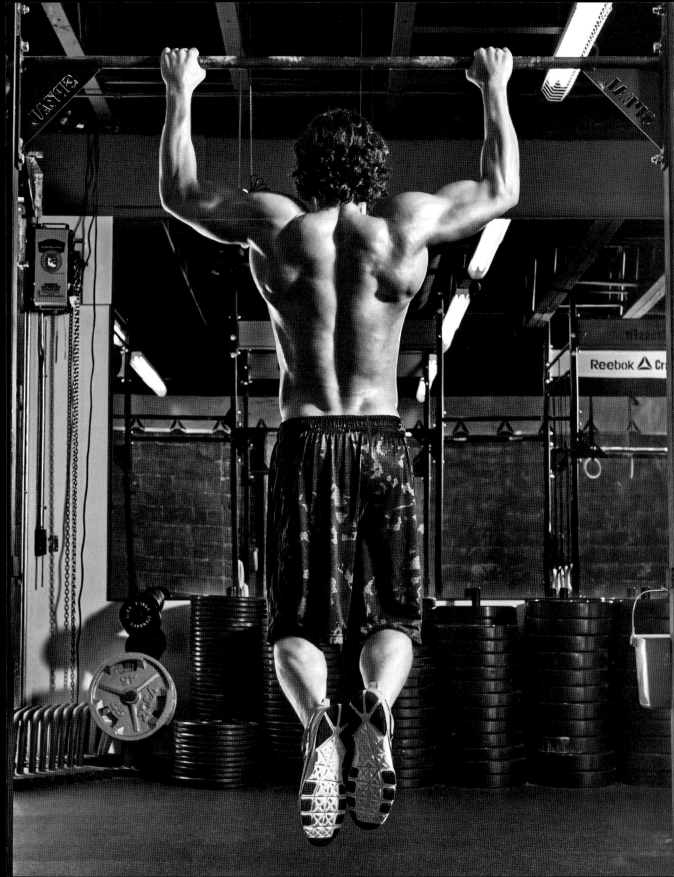

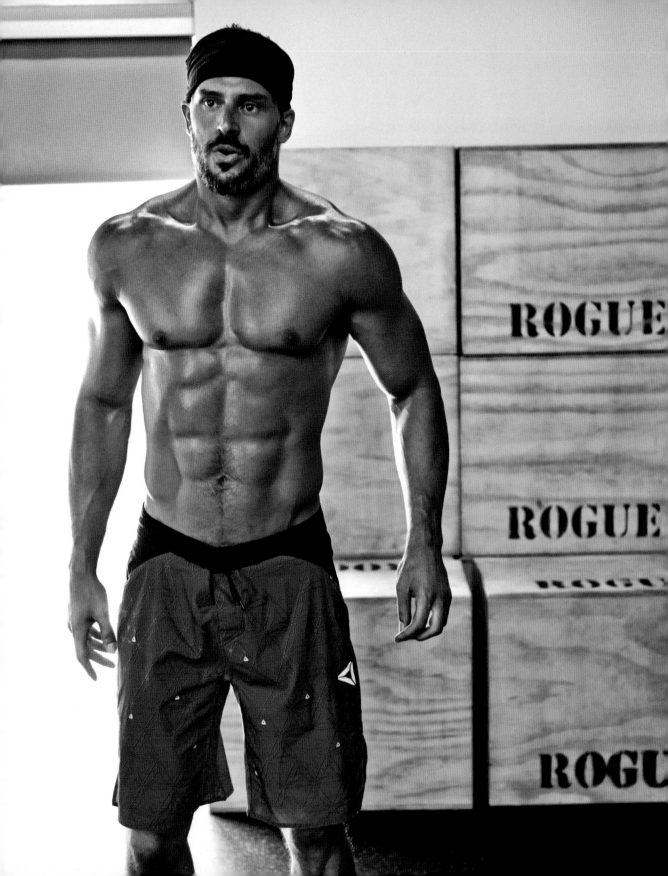

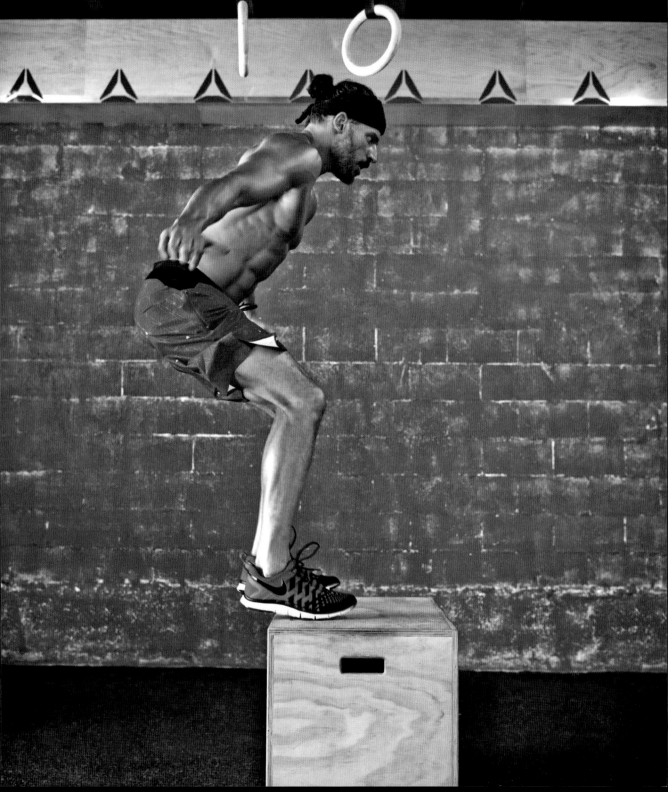

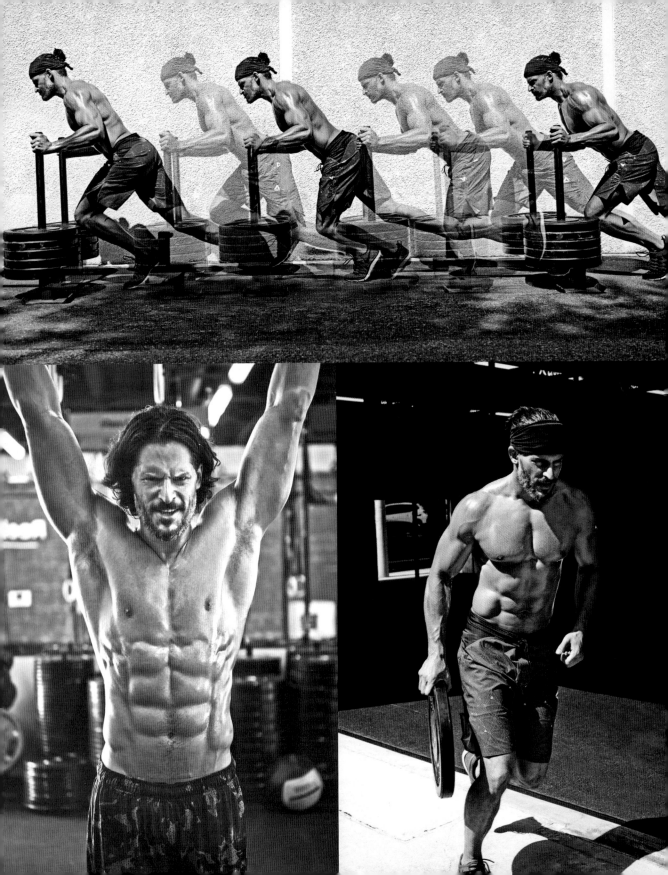

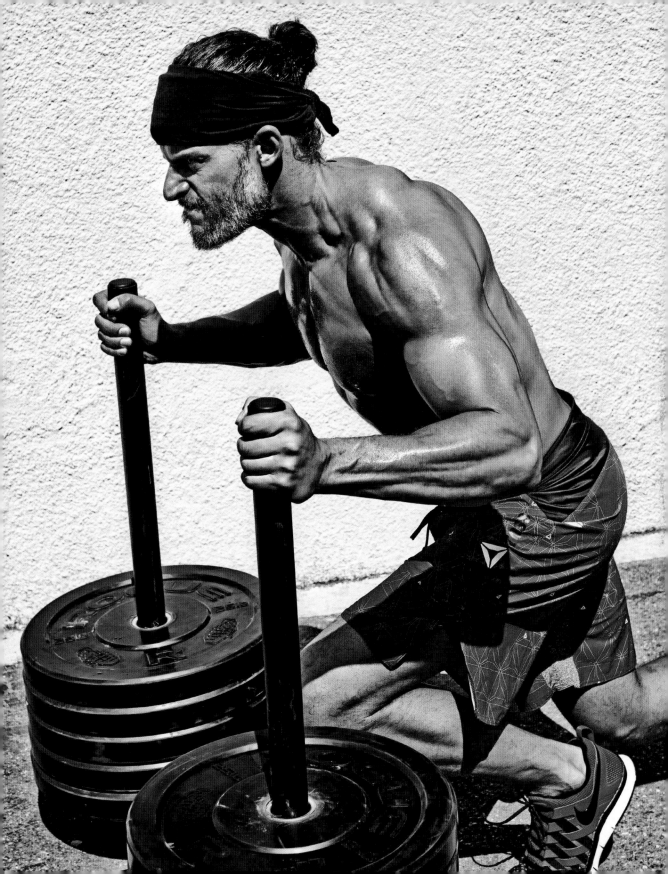

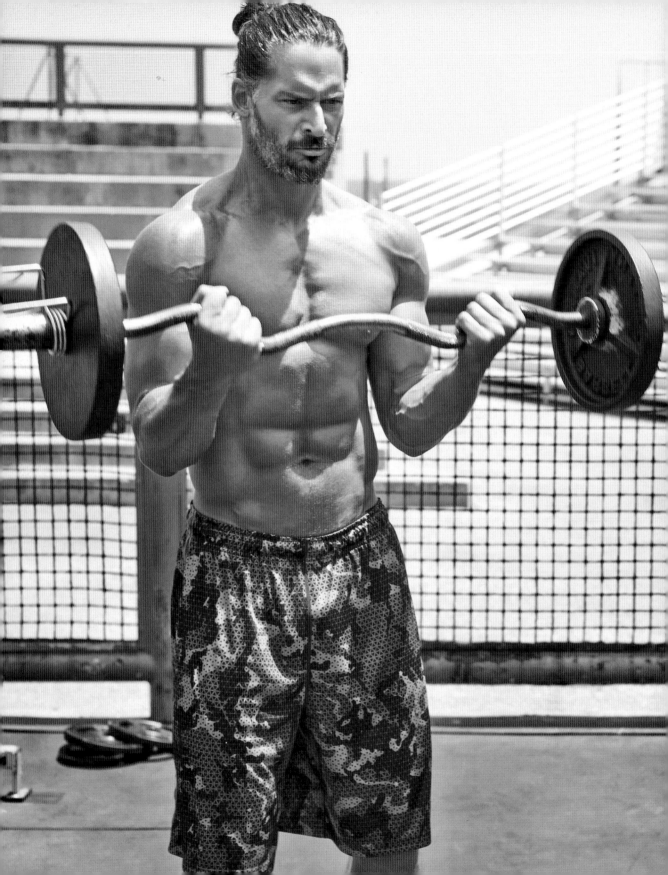

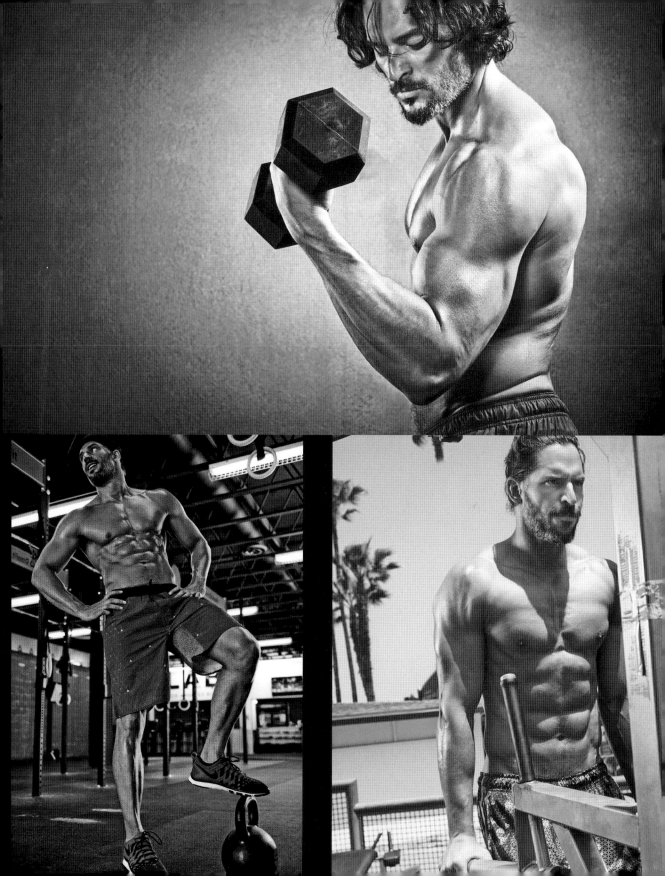

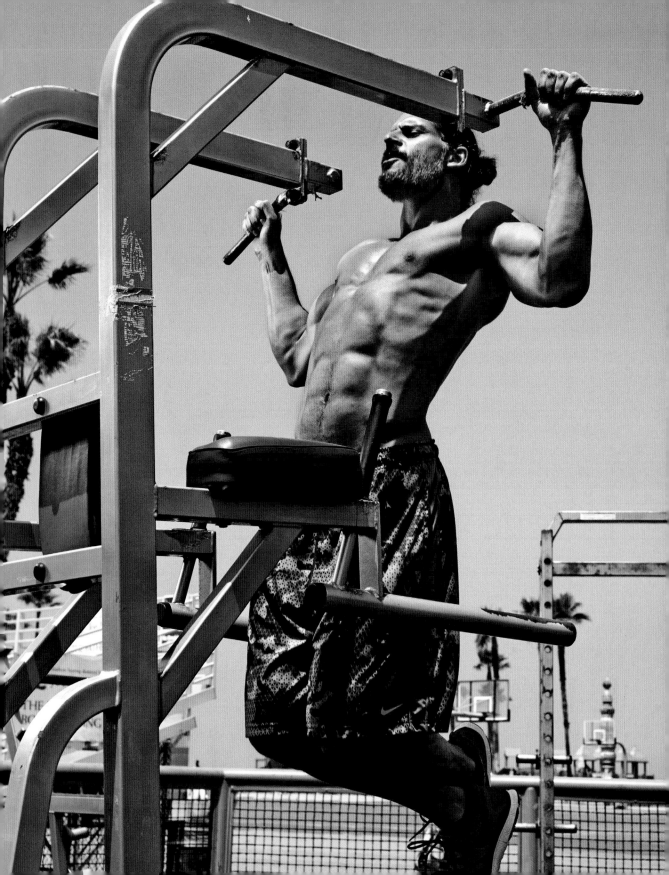

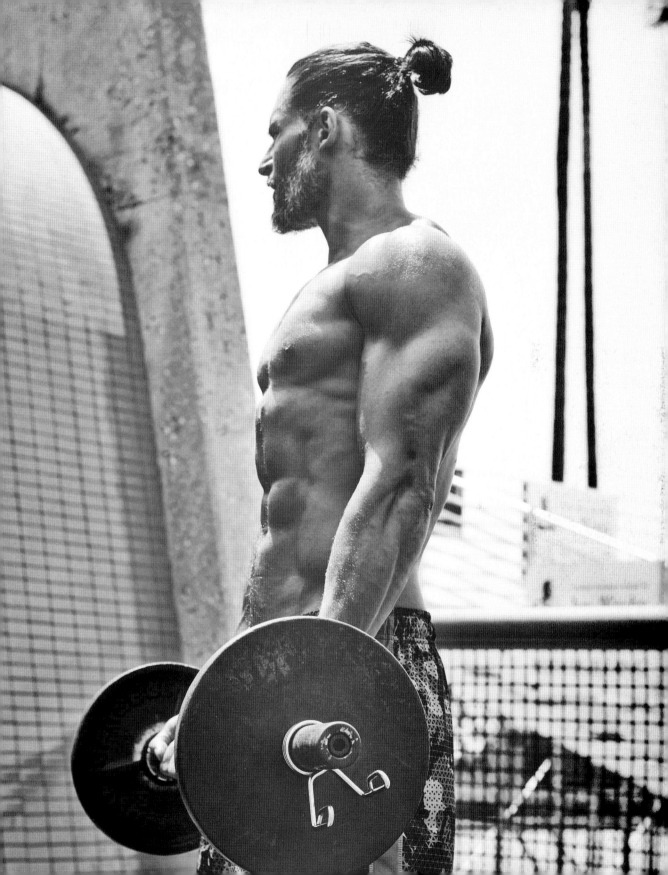

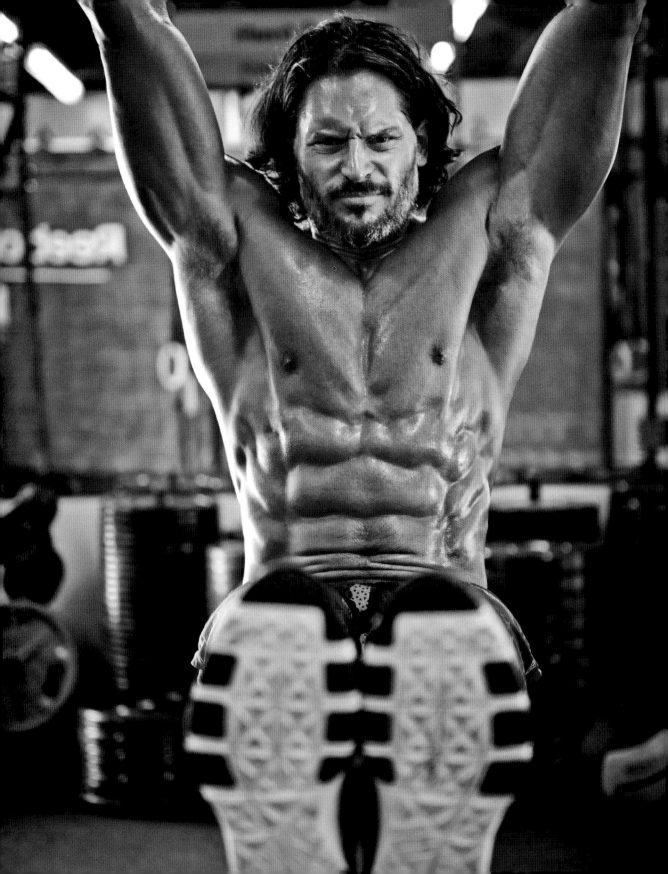

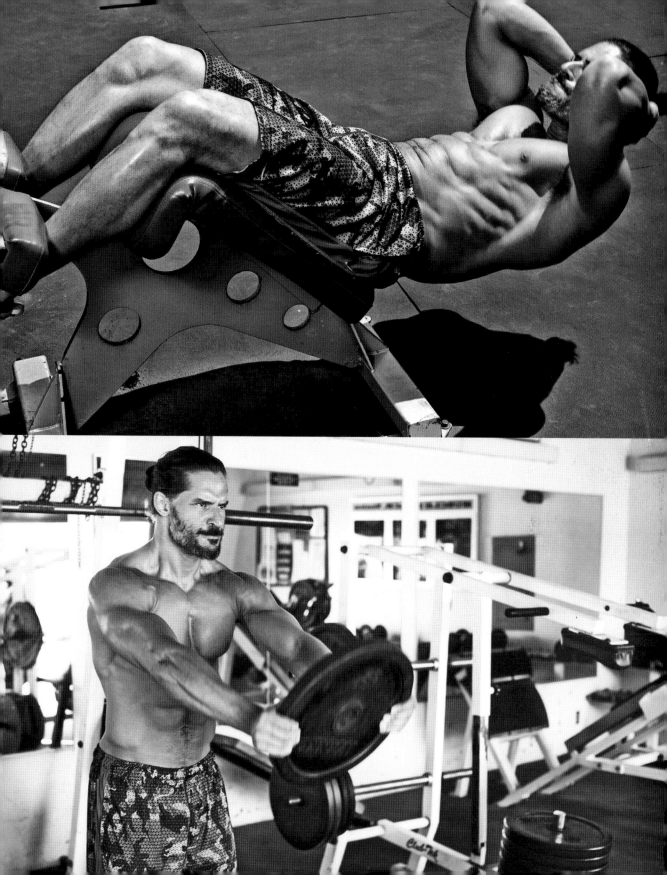

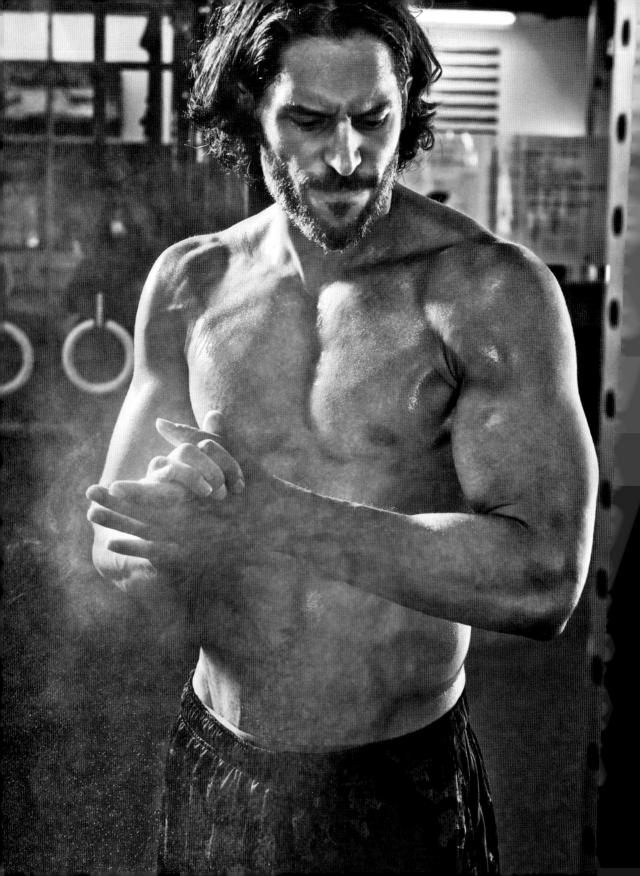

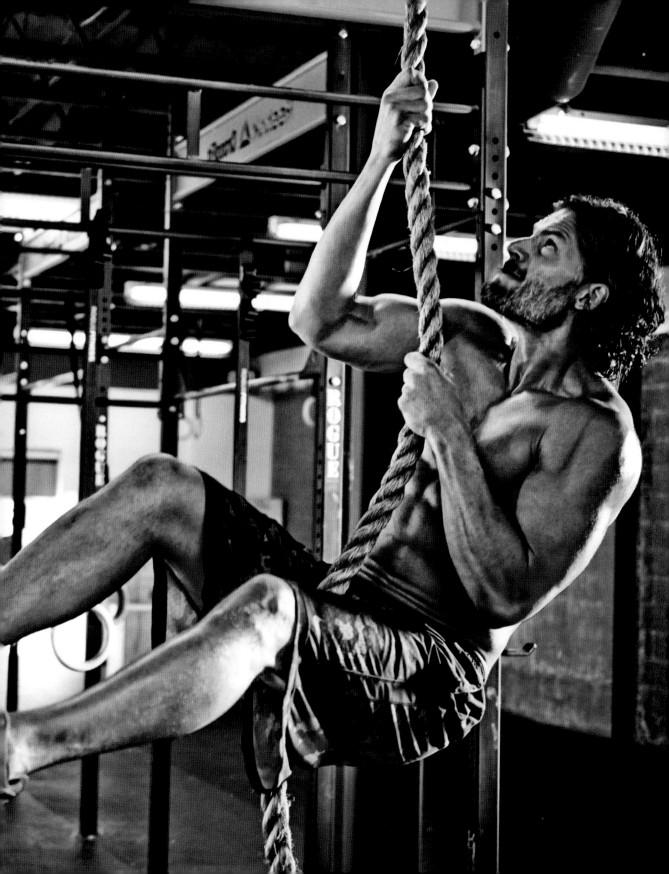

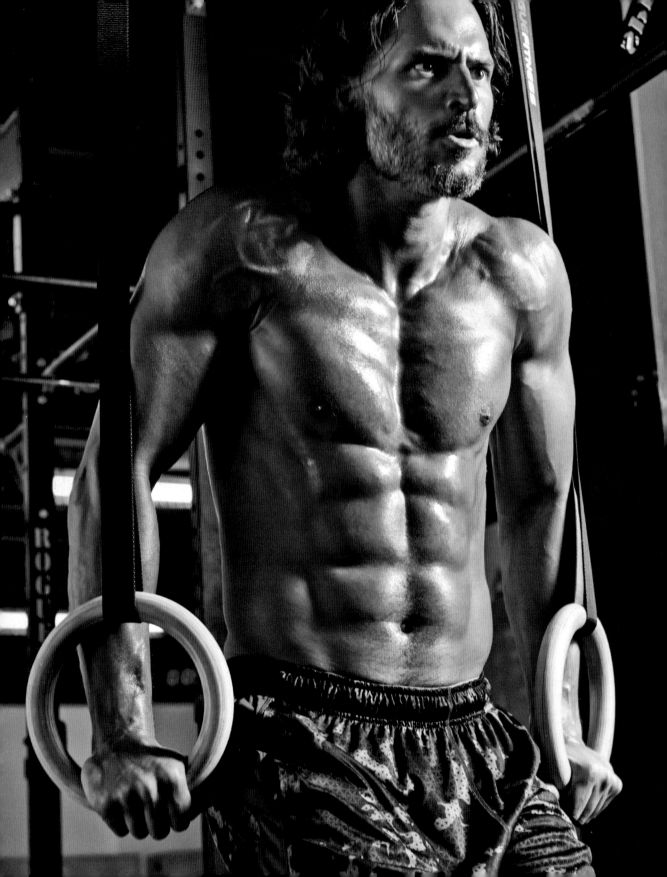

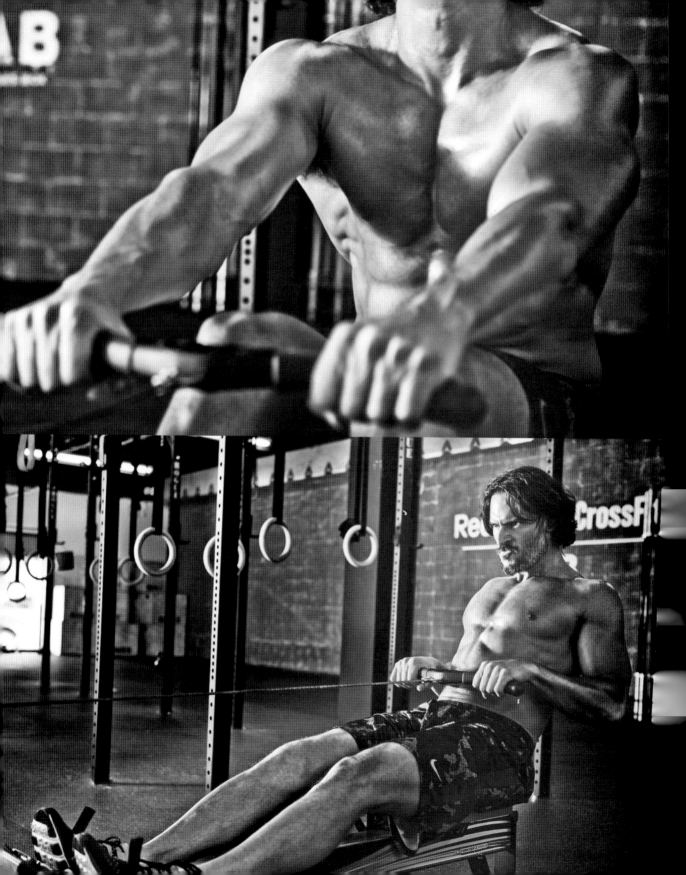

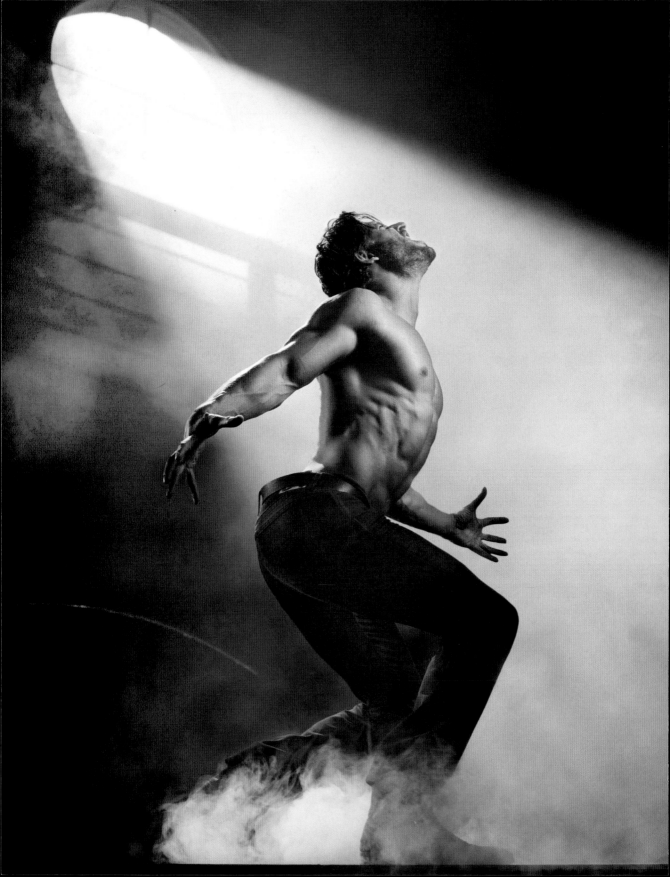

What I'm doing now in terms of working out would never be possible if I were still just trying to get by. It's all footwork, knowledge, hard work, a healthy diet, and as close to eight hours of sleep as I can get, in order to avoid melting down on those around me.

I had to figure out all of this on my own, the hard way. But the good news is, now you don't.

MAN UP

I want to think that we're in a progressive, understanding society, but the more I listen and observe, the more I realize most people are still incredibly misinformed. I see the influence of Joe Weider's social revolution around me in the coolers full of protein drinks at gas stations, on the racks and racks of fitness books and muscle magazines at newsstands, in the gyms on every corner, and in every high school and junior high. I *want* to believe we're health conscious, but I still see so much confusion and division. There is a huge chasm that needs to be closed, in order for us all to move forward together.

I leave you as the appointed torchbearer to spread Evolution. Just as Arnold has asked me to take on his mission of fitness and push it forward, I need your help. I challenge you to first transform your body, using what's in this book, and then be the spark that makes others want to change, as well. A long time ago, Dr. Jim Mooney and his lab rats lit a fire in me to change. I can only hope that my story inspires and motivates you to become what you were meant to be.

You might feel like you should be farther along than you are, and that's okay. I've certainly felt that way, and the memory of that feeling is exactly what motivates me now. I know that I still have a long way to go. So don't get frustrated; let's see where you are in six weeks. In six months. In a year.

I didn't fill out until my late twenties. It just wasn't happening—until it did. It was harder doing this naturally. I watched the kids around me on the high school football team experimenting with steroids, and as much as I wanted to win, I wanted to do it my way. It makes me sad to think back to a couple of those guys experimenting with other drugs in addition to the steroids, who wound up dead of overdoses a few years out of high school. I also don't see the need to hit up an antiaging clinic if you do this the right way. It just takes more discipline. Your body won't help you unless you help it and never stop.

In hindsight, there were so many "God fingerprints" all over my life that in a way, it seems like I've merely been a willing passenger on this incredible adventure . . . like it was all meant to be. For example, I believe that I was meant to meet Ron. He, like me, was the guy who couldn't do one pull-up or one dip in high school. Ron was the guy who couldn't bench the bar. Yet here we are being asked to lead the way into the future of fitness. A couple of guys who wove our endless struggles and difficulties into technique and inspiration.

Stop trying to figure out what you can get away with. Your new mantra is *"What can I become?"*

Find your reason to train and evolve.

As for the haters, they'll be there to let you know that you're doing something right. Forget them. They'll either join the movement and change or go down with their own sinking ship, the SS *Self-Loathing*.

When all is said and done, you won't regret the struggle, the fight, the sweat, or the image you see in the mirror. All you'll remember is the journey and the transformation. You'll look back with pride at how you looked into the mirror, wanted something more for yourself, and decided to get up and do something about it. You'll be reminded every day of how you smashed through every wall and mental barrier placed in your way and set no limits on what you could become . . . on *who* you could become.

Your past is the pedestal. It's waiting for you to place the statue on top.

What's your statue going to be?

CHAPTER 11

Exercise
Descriptions

CHEST

BARBELL BENCH PRESS

1. Grasp a barbell with an overhand grip that's just wider than shoulder width, and hold it above your sternum, with your arms completely straight.

2. Lower the bar straight down in a controlled fashion. Make sure you keep your elbows tucked in close to your body, so that your upper arms form a 45-degree angle to your body in the down position.

3. Pause, and then press the bar in a straight line back up to the starting position.

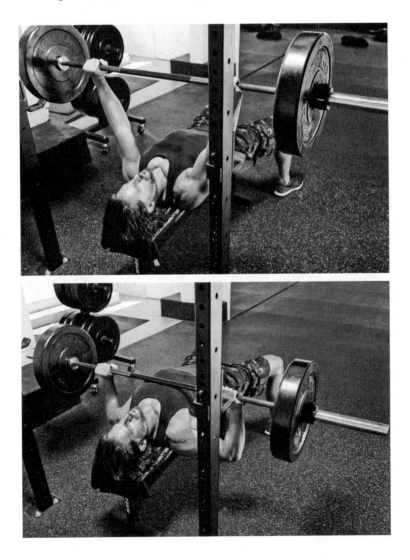

DUMBBELL BENCH PRESS

1. Lie flat on a bench. Grab a pair of dumbbells and lie faceup on the bench.

2. Hold the dumbbells directly above your shoulders, with your arms straight. Lower the dumbbells to the sides of your chest.

3. Pause, and then press the weights back above your chest.

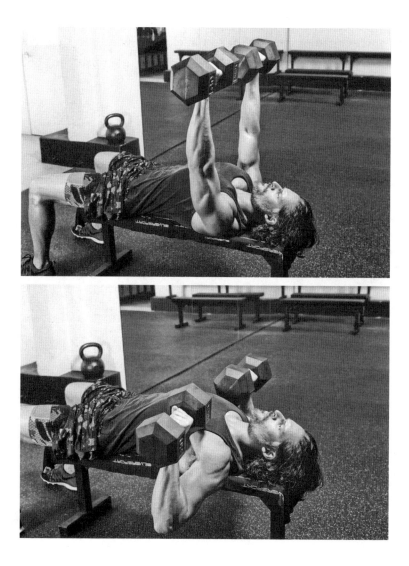

BARBELL INCLINE PRESS

1. Position your body on an incline bench that's angled at about 30 degrees to 45 degrees.

2. Grab a barbell with an overhand grip that's just wider than shoulder width and hold it above your sternum, with your arms straight.

3. Lower the bar straight down.

4. Pause, and then press the bar in a straight line back up to the starting position. Make sure you keep your elbows tucked in close to your body, so that in the down position your upper arms form a 45-degree angle with your body.

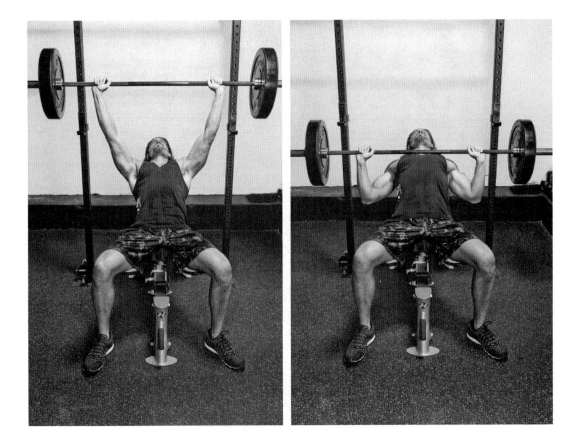

DUMBBELL INCLINE PRESS

1. Set an adjustable bench to an incline of 30 degrees to 45 degrees. Grab a pair of dumbbells and lie faceup on the bench.

2. Hold the dumbbells directly above your shoulders, with your arms straight. Lower the dumbbells to the sides of your chest.

3. Pause, and then press the weights back above your chest.

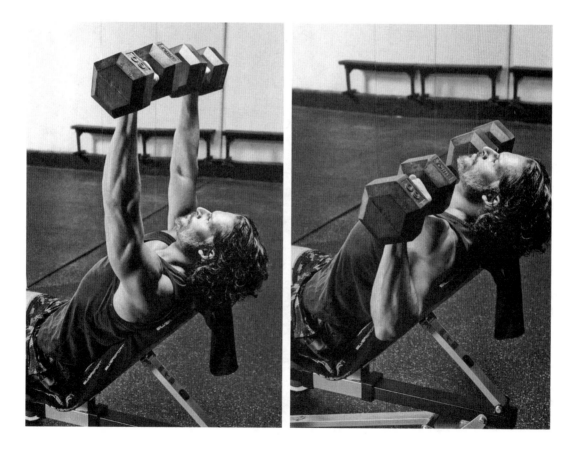

PEC DECK

1. Adjust the seat of the Pec Deck machine so that the handles out to your sides are just below shoulder level. Sit so that your back is upright against the rest, with your feet flat on the floor.

2. Grab hold of the handles and arch your back slightly, sticking out your chest.

3. Squeeze your chest, bringing together your hands. Pause for 1 second.

4. Return to the starting position and repeat until you complete the prescribed reps.

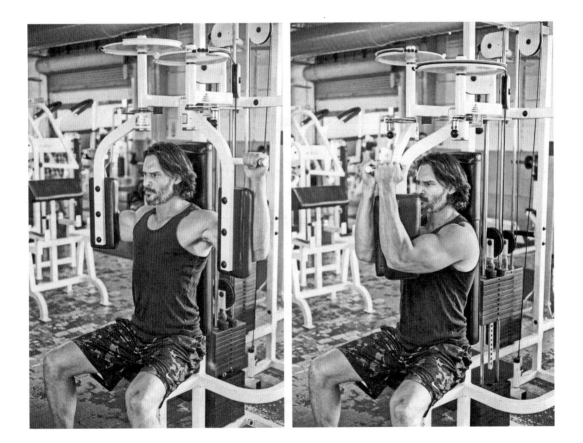

DUMBBELL FLYE

1. Grab a pair of dumbbells and lie on your back on a flat bench.

2. Raise your arms straight above your chest, with your palms facing each other and your elbows slightly bent.

3. Slowly lower the dumbbells in an arc down and away from your body.

4. Once the dumbbells are almost in-line with your chest, reverse the movement back to the starting position, making sure to squeeze the muscles in your chest at the top of the movement.

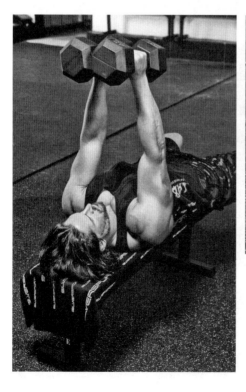
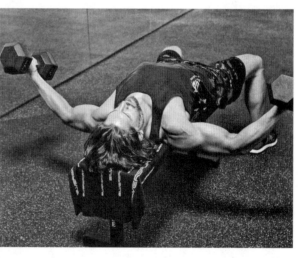

CLOSE-GRIP BARBELL BENCH PRESS

1. Grasp a barbell with an overhand grip that has your hands a few inches apart, and hold it above your sternum, with your arms completely straight.

2. Lower the bar straight down in a controlled fashion. Make sure you keep your elbows tucked in close to your body, so that your upper arms form a 45-degree angle to your body in the down position.

3. Pause, and then press the bar in a straight line back up to the starting position.

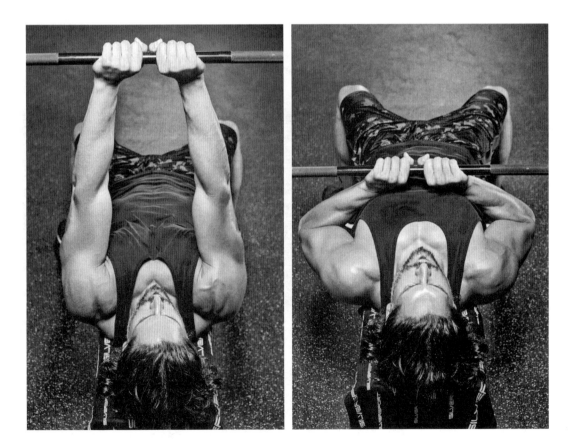

BAR DIP

1. Hoist yourself up on parallel bars, with your torso perpendicular to the floor. You'll maintain this posture throughout the exercise. Bend your knees and cross your ankles.

2. Slowly lower your body until your shoulder joints are below your elbows.

3. Push back up until your elbows are nearly straight but not locked.

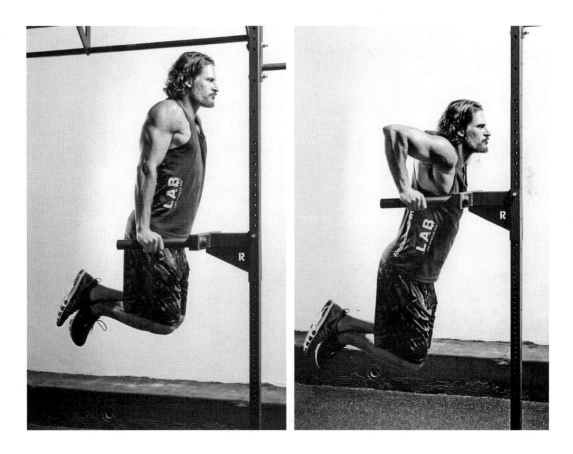

CABLE CHEST FLYE

1. Grab a pair of D-handles at the cable station and assume a staggered stance. Your arms should be extended straight in front of your chest, with your palms facing each other and your elbows slightly bent.

2. Slowly move your arms in an arc to the sides of your body.

3. Once the handles are almost in-line with your chest, reverse the movement back to the starting position, making sure to squeeze the muscles in your chest at the top of the movement.

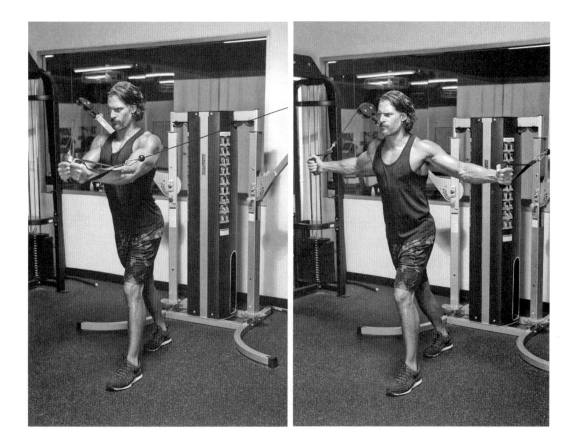

PUSH-UP

1. Get in a plank position and place your hands slightly wider than your shoulders. Your body should form a straight line from your ankles to your shoulders.

2. Squeeze your abs as tight as possible and keep them contracted for the entire exercise.

3. Lower your body until your chest nearly touches the floor, making sure to tuck your elbows close to the sides of your torso.

4. Pause, and then push yourself back to the starting position.

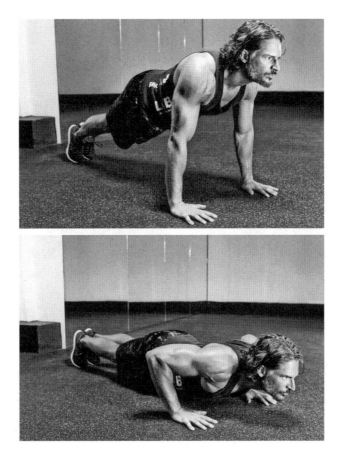

BENCH PLYO PUSH-UP

1. Assume a push-up position, with your hands on a bench, hands slightly wider than your shoulders. Your body should form a straight line from your ankles to your head.

2. Bend your elbows and lower your body until your chest nearly touches the bench.

3. Then, bench-press yourself up so explosively that your hands leave the bench.

4. Land, reset your body, and repeat.

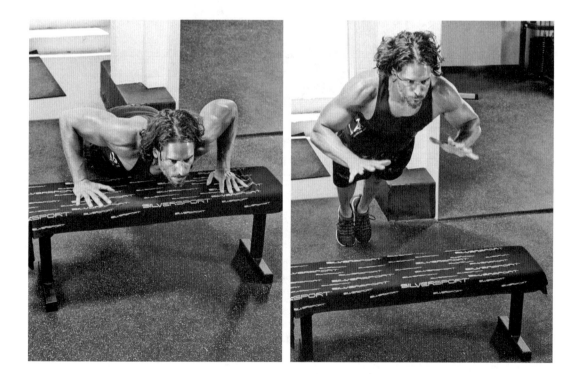

BENCH PUSH-UP

1. Assume a push-up position, with your hands on a bench, slightly wider than your shoulders. Your body should form a straight line from your ankles to your head. Squeeze your abs as tight as possible and keep them contracted for the entire exercise.

2. Lower your body until your chest nearly touches the bench, making sure to tuck your elbows close to the sides of your torso.

3. Pause, and then push yourself back to the starting position.

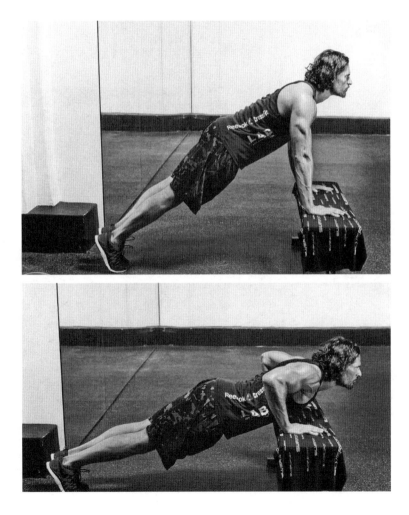

NARROW-GRIP BENCH PUSH-UP

1. Place your hands on a bench, narrower than your shoulders, with your legs and feet straight behind you. Your body should form a straight line from your ankles to your head. Squeeze your abs as tight as possible and keep them contracted for the entire exercise.

2. Lower your body until your chest nearly touches the bench, making sure to tuck your elbows close to the sides of your torso.

3. Pause, and then push yourself back to the starting position.

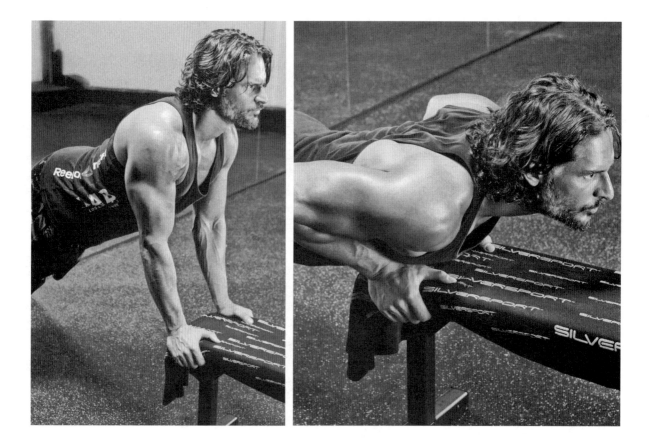

PLYO PUSH-UP OVER A PLATE

1. Begin in push-up position with one hand on a weight plate and the other on the floor. Lower your body to perform a push-up.

2. Press up explosively so that both arms leave the floor, and then land with your opposite hand on the plate and your other hand on the floor.

3. Lower your body and repeat, this time doing a plyo push-up back to the starting position.

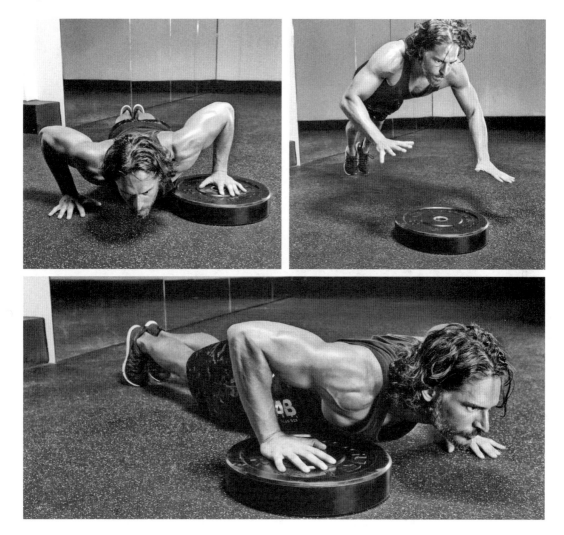

LAT PULL-DOWN WITH WIDE PRONATED GRIP

1. Sit at a lat pull-down station and grab the bar with an overhand grip that's just wider than shoulder width. Your arms should be completely straight and your torso upright.

2. Pull your shoulder blades down and back, and bring the bar to your chest.

3. Pause, and then return to the starting position.

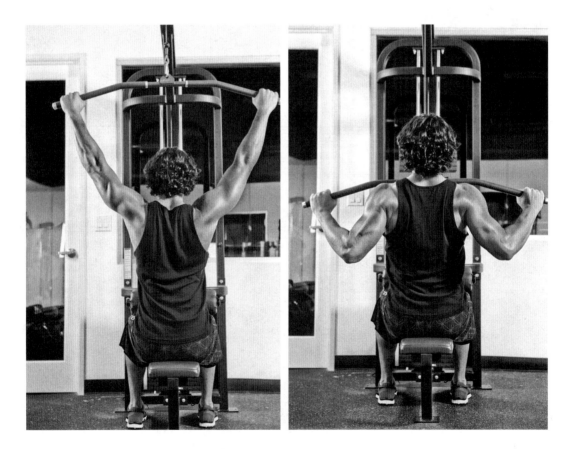

LAT PULL-DOWN WITH WIDE NEUTRAL GRIP

1. Sit at a lat pull-down station and grab the bar with a neutral grip that's just wider than shoulder width, so that your palms are facing each other. Your arms should be completely straight and your torso upright.

2. Pull your shoulder blades down and back, and bring the bar to your chest.

3. Pause, and then return to the starting position.

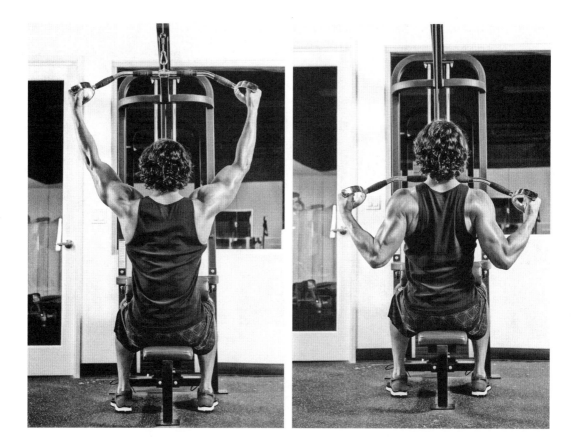

LAT PULL-DOWN WITH NARROW NEUTRAL GRIP

1. Sit at a lat pull-down station and grab the handles. Your arms should be completely straight and your torso upright.

2. Pull your shoulder blades down and back, and bring the handle to your chest.

3. Pause, and then return to the starting position.

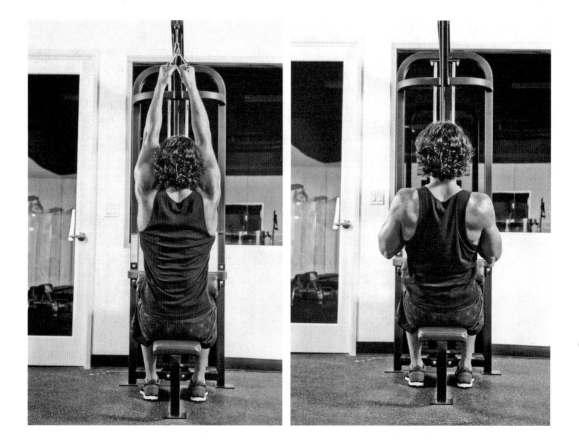

LAT PULL-DOWN WITH NARROW SUPINATED GRIP

1. Sit at a lat pull-down station and grab the bar with an underhand grip that's about shoulder-width apart. Your arms should be completely straight and your torso upright.

2. Pull your shoulder blades down and back, and bring the bar to your chest.

3. Pause, and then return to the starting position.

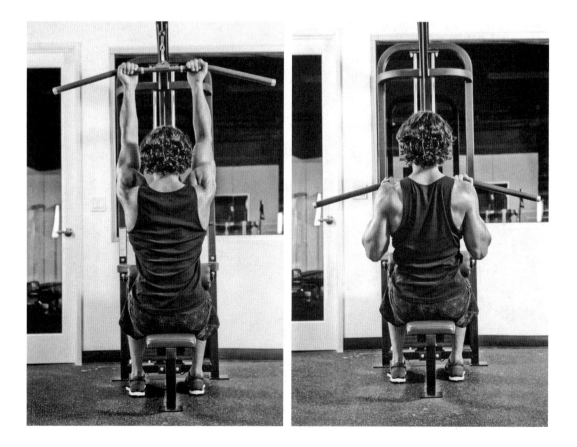

ONE-ARM DUMBBELL ROW WITH NEUTRAL GRIP

1. Grab a dumbbell in one hand, with your palm facing inward toward your torso, and place your other hand on the bench.

2. Bend at your hips (don't round your lower back) and lower your torso until it's almost parallel to the floor. Let the dumbbell hang at arm's length.

3. Without moving your torso, row the dumbbell upward by raising your upper arms, bending your elbows, and squeezing together your shoulder blades.

4. Pause, and then lower the dumbbell back to the starting position.

5. Do all reps, switch the dumbbell to your other hand, and repeat.

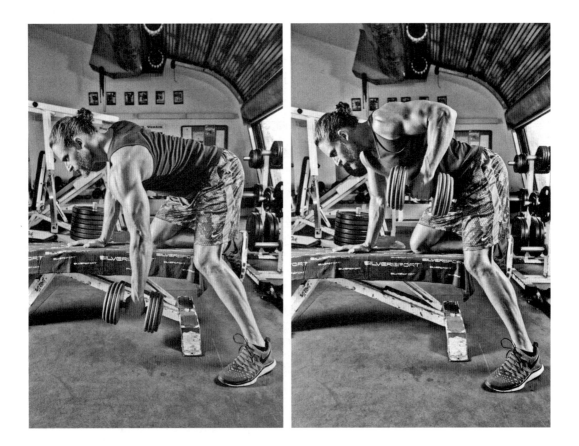

ONE-ARM DUMBBELL ROW WITH SUPINATED GRIP

1. Grab a dumbbell in one hand with an underhand grip, so that your palm faces forward, and place your other hand on the bench.

2. Bend at your hips (don't round your lower back) and lower your torso until it's almost parallel to the floor. Let the dumbbell hang at arm's length.

3. Without moving your torso, row the dumbbell upward by raising your upper arms, bending your elbows, and squeezing together your shoulder blades.

4. Pause, and then lower the dumbbell back to the starting position.

5. Do all reps, switch the dumbbell to your other hand, and repeat.

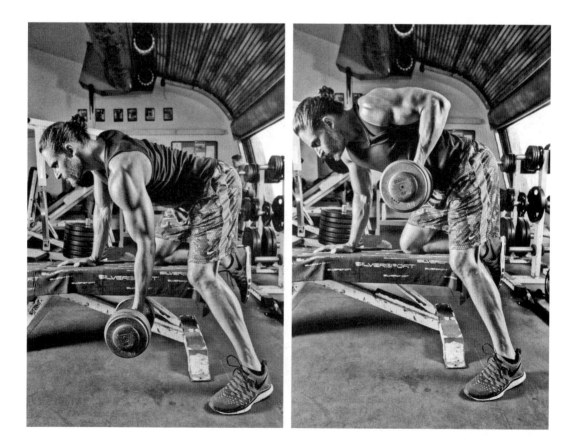

TWO-ARM BENT-OVER DUMBBELL ROW WITH NEUTRAL GRIP

1. Holding a dumbbell in each hand, stand with your feet shoulder-width apart.

2. Bend the knees slightly and bend over at the waist, with your back straight. Avoid rounding the upper back and keep the head neutral. Extend your arms fully so that each dumbbell is just above the floor.

3. Contract your back and pull both dumbbells up to your rib cage. Be sure to pull through the elbow and hold for 1 second in the top position.

4. Lower the dumbbell to the fully extended arm position and repeat.

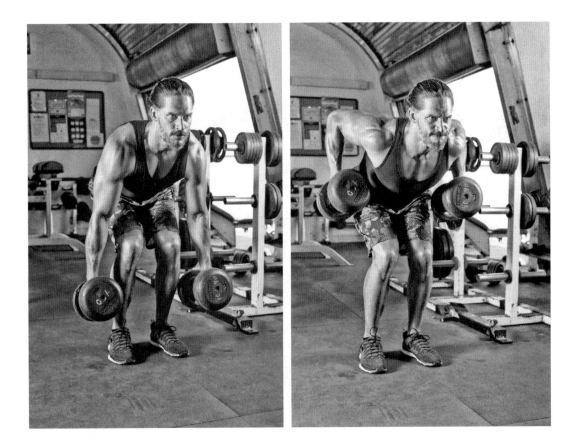

LOW ROW WITH WIDE PRONATED GRIP

1. Attach a straight bar to the cable and position yourself with your feet braced.

2. Position your hands about 1½ times shoulder-width apart.

3. With your knees slightly bent, sit up straight, push your chest out, and pull your shoulders down and back. Without moving your torso and keeping your core braced, pull the bar to your lower chest.

4. Pause, then slowly return the weight to the starting position.

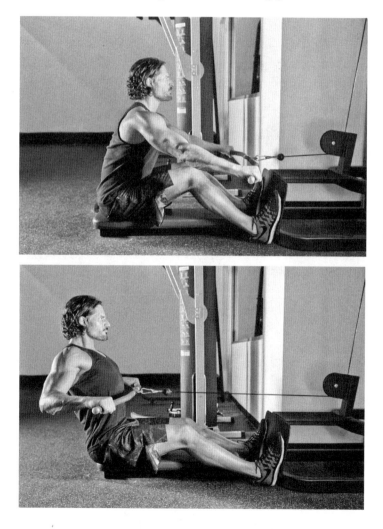

LOW ROW WITH WIDE NEUTRAL GRIP

1. Attach a long bar with handles to the cable and position yourself with your feet braced. Position your hands about 1½ times shoulder-width apart with your palms facing each other.

2. With your knees slightly bent, sit up straight, push your chest out, and pull your shoulders down and back. Without moving your torso and keeping your core braced, pull the bar to your lower chest.

3. Pause, then slowly return the weight to the starting position.

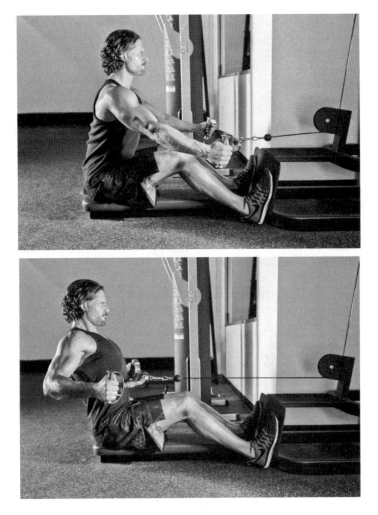

LOW ROW WITH NARROW SUPINATED GRIP

1. Attach a straight bar to the cable and position yourself with your feet braced. Hold the bar with an underhand grip and position your hands closer than shoulder-width apart.

2. With your knees slightly bent, sit up straight, push your chest out, and pull your shoulders down and back. Without moving your torso and keeping your core braced, pull the bar to your lower chest.

3. Pause, then slowly return the weight to the starting position.

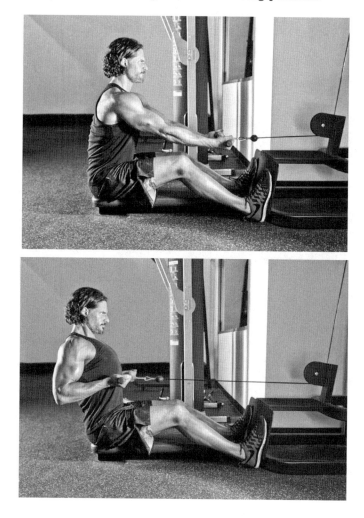

LOW ROW WITH NARROW NEUTRAL GRIP

1. Attach a V-bar (or stirrup grip) to the cable and position yourself with your feet braced. Grab the attachment with your palms facing each other.

2. Without moving your torso and keeping your core braced, pull the bar to your lower chest.

3. Pause, then slowly return the weight to the starting position.

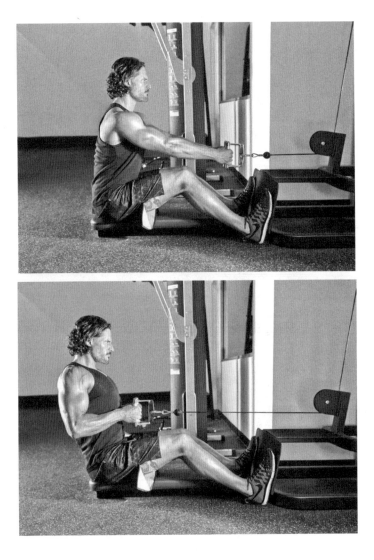

PULL-UP WITH WIDE PRONATED GRIP

1. Grab a chin-up bar with a wide overhand grip.

2. Hang at arm's length and pull your shoulder blades down and back so that your shoulders are as far from your ears as possible.

3. Pull your chest to the bar as you squeeze together your shoulder blades.

4. Pause, and then lower your body back to a dead hang.

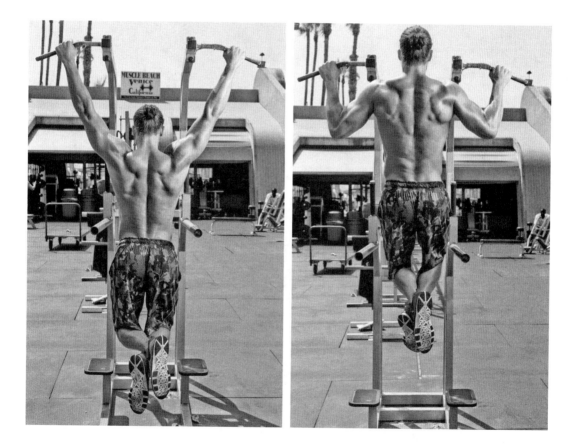

CHIN-UP WITH NARROW SUPINATED GRIP

1. Grab a chin-up bar with a narrow underhand grip.

2. Hang at arm's length and pull your shoulder blades down and back so that your shoulders are as far from your ears as possible.

3. Pull your chest to the bar as you squeeze together your shoulder blades.

4. Pause, and then lower your body back to the starting position.

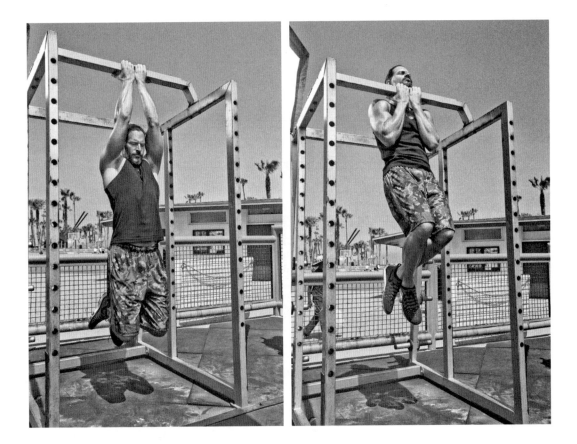

BENT-OVER BARBELL ROW WITH WIDE PRONATED GRIP

1. Grab a barbell with an overhand grip, with your hands wider than shoulder-width apart.

2. Hold the bar at arm's length, and then bend at your hips and lower your torso until it's almost parallel to the floor. Your knees should be slightly bent and your lower back arched naturally.

3. Squeeze your shoulder blades together and pull the bar up to your upper abs.

4. Pause, and then return the bar to the starting position.

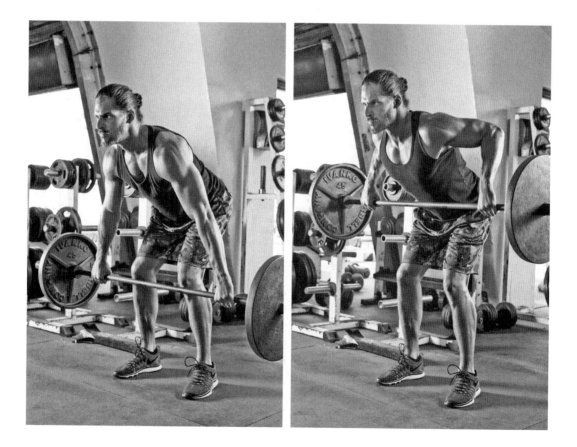

BENT-OVER SUPINATED LOW CABLE ROW

1. Attach a straight-bar attachment to the cable machine and position your body with your feet braced.

2. Grab the attachment with a narrow underhand grip, bend your knees slightly, and position your torso at a 45-degree angle, with your shoulders down and back.

3. Without moving your torso, pull the bar toward your upper abs.

4. Pause, and then return to the starting position.

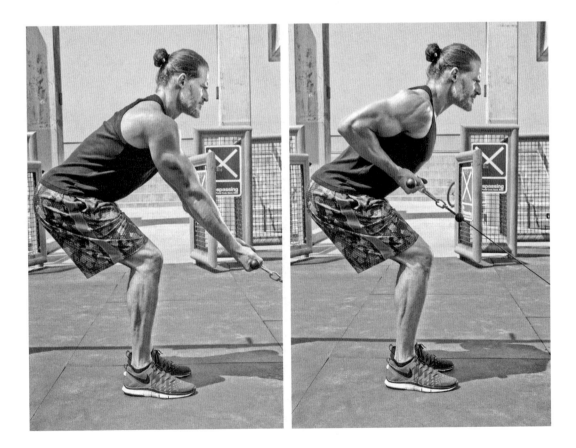

BARBELL PULL-OVER

1. Sitting on a flat bench, hold a barbell in your lap with both hands.

2. Lie back on the bench and lift the barbell directly overhead, with your arms fully extended and your triceps locked. This is your starting position. You may also have a partner hand you the barbell in the starting position.

3. Bend the elbows, then lower the weight until the barbell is behind your head and your elbows are beside your head. You should feel an intense stretch in your triceps and lats.

4. Pause for one second in the bottom position and then return to the starting position by contracting the triceps and lats.

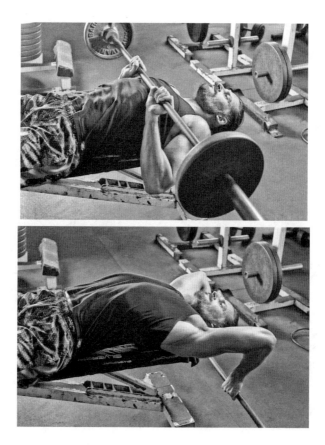

SEATED DUMBBELL ROW

1. Grab a pair of dumbbells and sit on the edge of a bench. Bend over slightly at your waist so that your torso forms a 45-degree angle to the floor. Your arms should hang at your sides and be perpendicular to the floor, with your palms facing your body.

2. Without moving your torso, pull both dumbbells up to your rib cage.

3. Pause, and then lower the dumbbells back to the starting position.

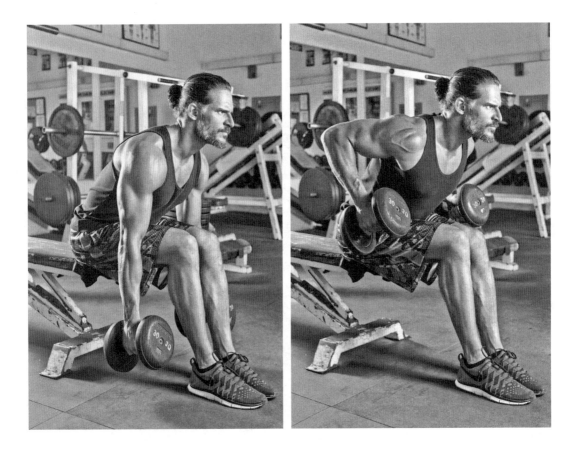

SEATED DUMBBELL SWIM AND ROW

1. Grab a pair of dumbbells and sit on the edge of a bench. Bend over slightly at your waist so that your torso forms a 45-degree angle to the floor.

2. Extend your arms out in from your torso until they are almost parallel to the floor, with your palms facing the floor. Without moving your torso, pull both dumbbells up to your rib cage by driving your elbows behind your back.

3. Pause, and then lower the dumbbells down and out and toward your ankles, and in one movement raise them back to the starting position and repeat.

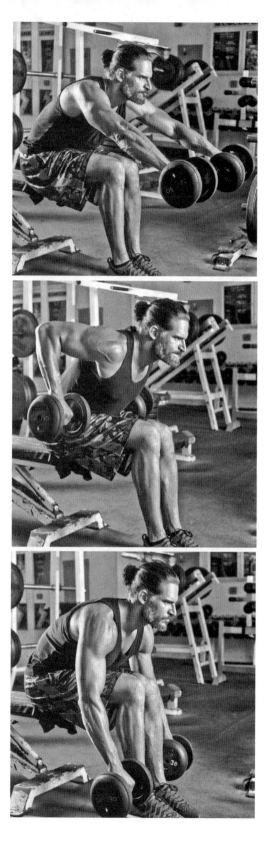

STANDING FRONT-LAT PUSH-DOWN

1. Stand at a lat pull-down station and grab the bar with an overhand grip that's about shoulder-width apart.

2. Keep your arms straight, elbows locked, and body upright, and pull down the bar toward your thighs.

3. Pause, and then reverse the motion back to the starting position.

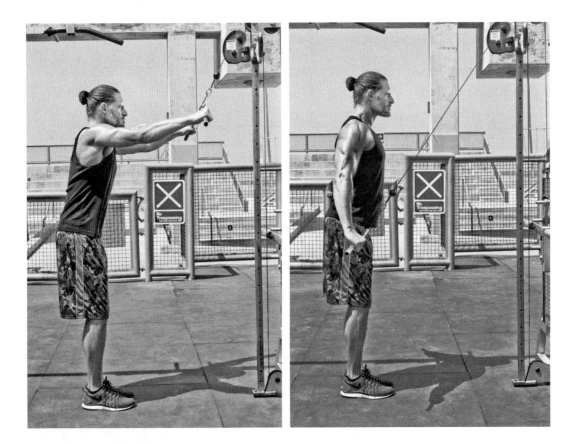

BARBELL BACK SQUAT

1. Hold a barbell across your upper back with an overhand grip and your feet shoulder-width apart.

2. Keeping your lower back arched, lower your body as deep as you can by pushing back your hips and bending your knees.

3. Pause, and then reverse the movement back to the starting position.

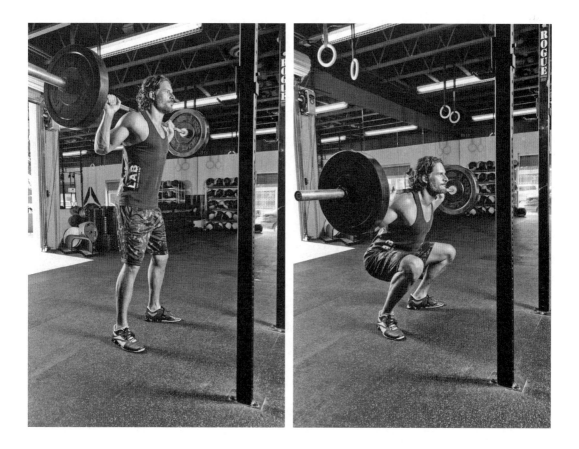

BARBELL FRONT SQUAT

1. Hold a barbell with an overhand grip that's just beyond shoulder width.

2. Raise your upper arms until they're parallel to the floor and allow the bar to rest on the front of your shoulders.

3. Lower your body until the tops of your thighs are at least parallel to the floor.

4. Pause, and then push your body back to the starting position.

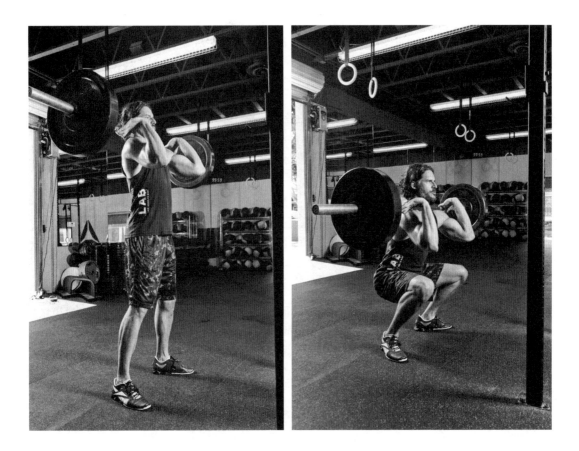

DEAD LIFT

1. Load a barbell and roll it up against your shins. Set your feet about shoulder-width apart.

2. Bend at your hips and knees, and grab the center of the bar with an overhand grip, your hands about 12 inches apart.

3. Without allowing your lower back to round, stand up, thrust your hips forward, and squeeze your glutes.

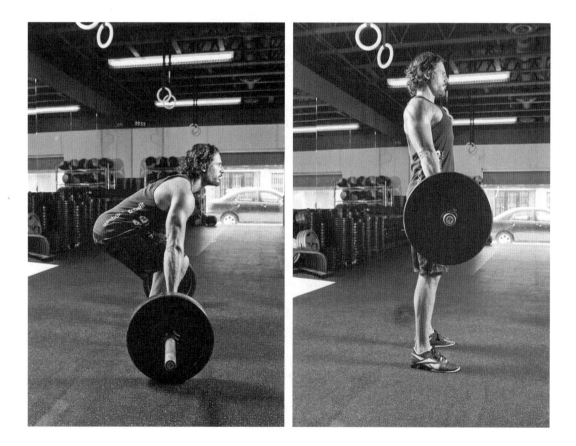

LEG PRESS

1. Sit in a leg press machine with your butt all the way back in the chair and your back flat against the chair. Place your feet on the platform roughly shoulder-width apart. Keep your heels flat.

2. Press the weighted platform away as you straighten your legs.

3. Return your legs to the starting position.

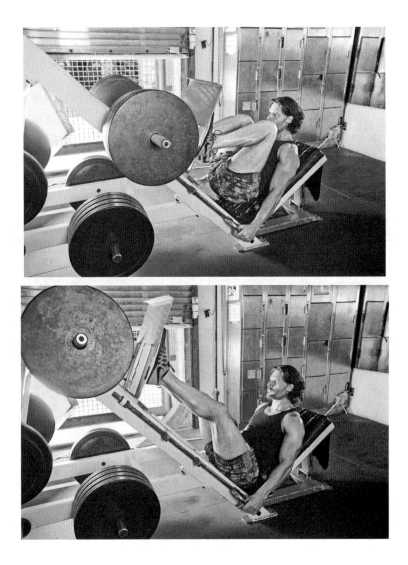

LEG CURL

1. Sit down on the machine and place your calves directly under the ankle pad.

2. Keeping your core tight, use your hamstrings to curl your ankles as close to your butt as possible.

3. Pause, and then slowly return the weight to the starting position.

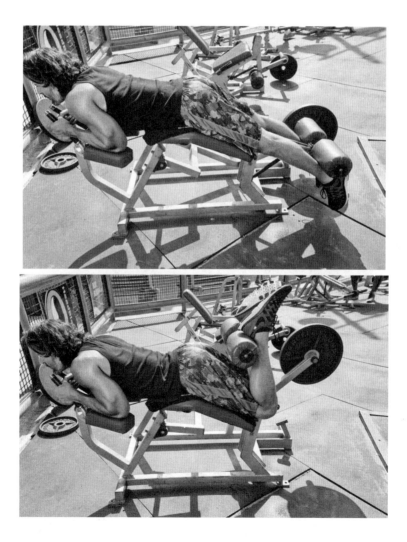

ONE-LEG LEG CURL

1. Sit down on the machine and place your calves directly under the ankle pad.

2. Keeping your core tight, use the hamstring of one leg to curl your ankle beneath you and as close to your butt as possible.

3. Pause, and then slowly return the weight to the starting position.

4. Perform for the prescribed number of repetitions and then repeat on the opposite leg.

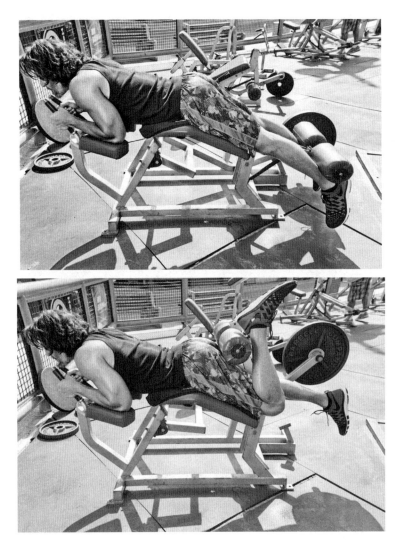

LEG EXTENSION

1. Sit in a knee extension machine with your knees bent at 90 degrees.

2. Extend both legs, lifting the leg pad upward. Straighten your knees at the top of the movement.

3. Lower the lower leg pad slowly. Return your legs to 90 degrees.

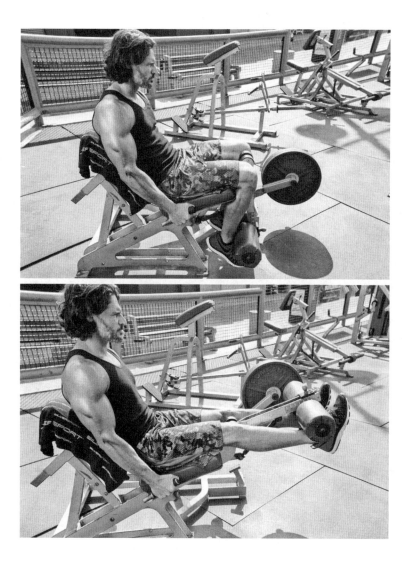

DUMBBELL OR KETTLEBELL GOBLET SQUAT

1. Hold a kettlebell or dumbbell vertically next to your chest, with both hands cupping one of the dumbbell plates.

2. Push back your hips and lower your body into a squat until your upper thighs are at least parallel to the floor. Your elbows should brush the insides of your knees in the bottom position.

3. Pause, and then press your body back up to the starting position.

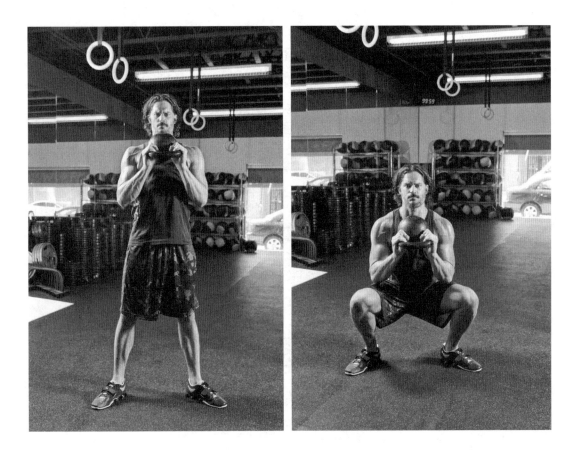

REVERSE LUNGE

1. Push out your chest and take a large step backward, lowering your rear knee toward the ground while keeping your front shin as vertical as possible.

2. Push yourself back to the starting position and repeat for the desired repetitions before switching legs.

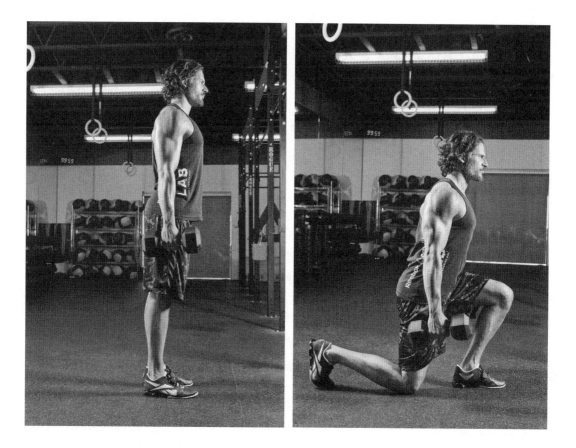

BULGARIAN SPLIT SQUAT

1. Grab a pair of dumbbells and hold them next to your sides, your palms facing each other. Stand in a staggered stance, your left foot in front of your right, and place your back foot on a bench.

2. Slowly lower your body as far as you can till your rear knee nearly touches the floor. Keep your torso as upright as possible and your lower back naturally arched.

3. Pause, then push yourself back up to the starting position as quickly as you can.

4. Complete the prescribed number of reps with your left leg forward, then do the same number with your right foot and your left on the bench.

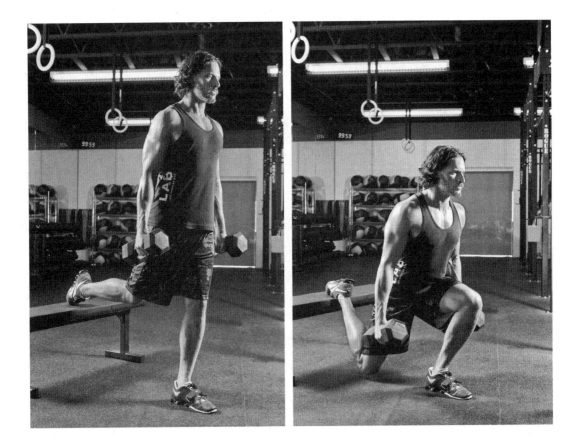

DUMBBELL BENCH STEP-UP

1. Grab a pair of dumbbells and hold them at your sides. Stand in front of a bench or step, and place your left foot firmly on the step.

2. Press your left heel into the step and push your body up until your left leg is straight.

3. Lower your body back down until your right foot touches the floor, and repeat.

4. Complete the prescribed number of repetitions with your left leg, and then do the same number with your right leg.

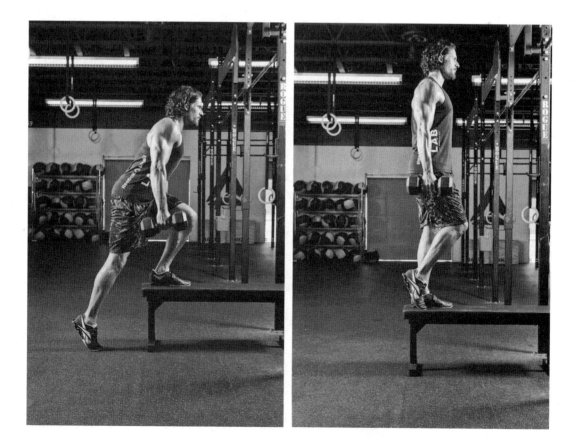

PLYO STEP-UP WITH A JUMP

1. Stand in front of a bench or step, and place your left foot firmly on the step. The step should be high enough that your knee is bent 90 degrees.

2. Press your left heel into the step and push your body up so that you jump into the air and swing your arms forward.

3. Land softly and return to the starting position.

4. Complete the prescribed number of repetitions with your left leg, then do the same number with your right leg.

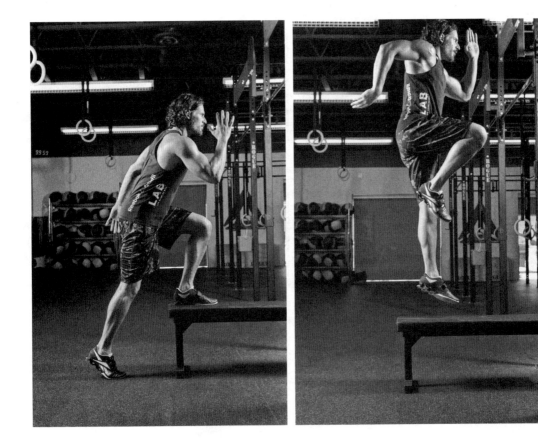

BODY-WEIGHT STEP-UP

1. Stand in front of a step or bench and place your left foot firmly on the step. The step should be high enough that your knee is bent 90 degrees.

2. Press your left heel into the step, and push your body up until your left leg is straight and you're standing on one leg on the step, keeping your right foot elevated.

3. Lower your body back down until your right foot touches the floor. Complete reps, then switch legs.

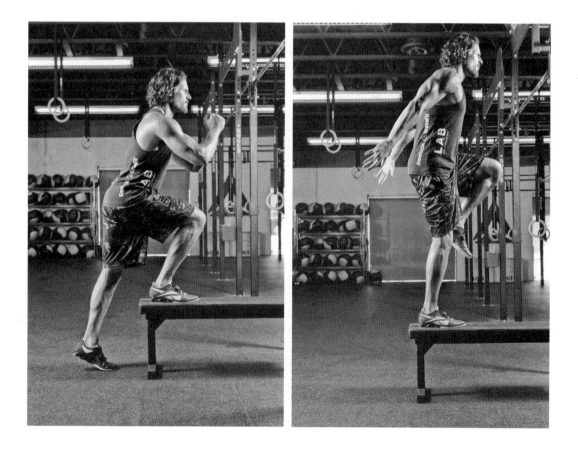

DUMBBELL WALKING LUNGE

1. Grab a pair of dumbbells and hold them at your sides, your palms facing each other. Stand tall with your feet hip-width apart, pull your shoulders back, and brace your core.

2. Step forward with one leg and slowly lower your body until your front knee is bent at least 90 degrees. Your rear knee should nearly touch the floor. Keep your torso as upright as possible and your lower back naturally arched.

3. Pause, then rise up and bring your back foot forward so that you move forward (like you're walking) and perform another lunge, but this time with your other leg.

4. Alternate the leg you step forward with each time.

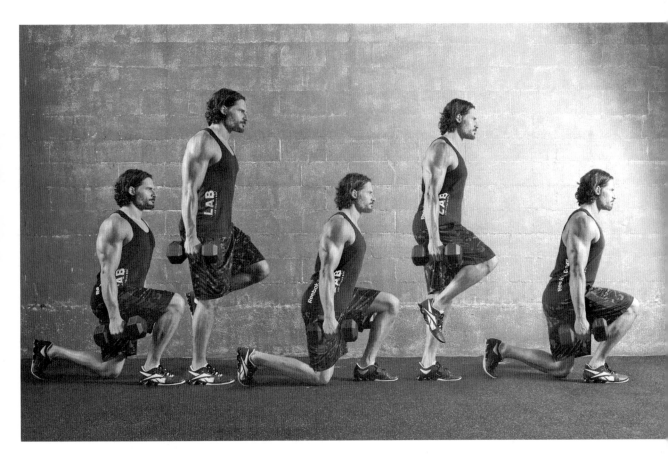

PLYO SQUAT JUMP

1. Dip your knees in preparation to leap, raising your arms straight in front of you.

2. Explosively jump as high as you can, swinging your arms back as you jump.

3. When you land, immediately squat down and jump again.

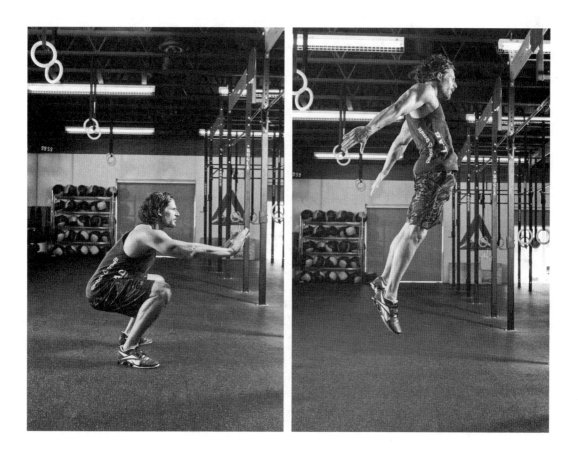

TRAVELING SQUAT JUMP

1. With your feet shoulder-width apart and your arms in front of you, lower your body by pushing your hips back and dipping your knees. Then, explode upward and forward and jump as far as you can, swinging your arms back.

2. Land softly in a quarter squat, reset, and repeat.

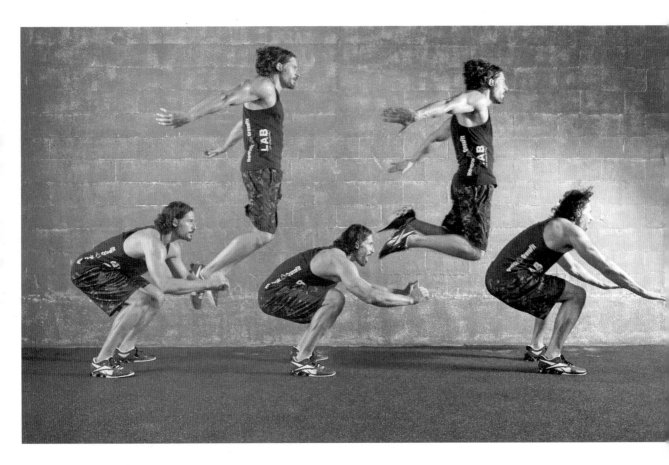

BODY-WEIGHT SQUAT

1. Stand as tall as you can, with your feet shoulder-width apart.

2. Lower your body as far as you can by pushing back your hips and bending your knees.

3. Pause, and then slowly push yourself back to the starting position.

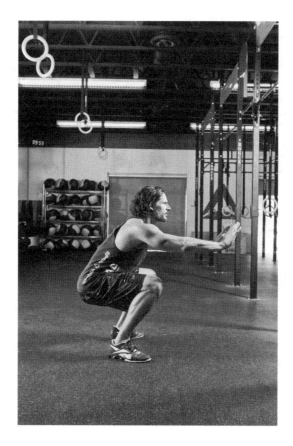

ONE-LEG LUNGE

1. Grab a pair of dumbbells and hold them at your sides, with your palms facing each other.

2. Step forward with your left leg and slowly lower your body until your front knee is bent at least 90 degrees.

3. Pause, and then push yourself back to the starting position as quickly as you can.

4. Complete the prescribed number of reps with your left leg, and then do the same number with your right leg.

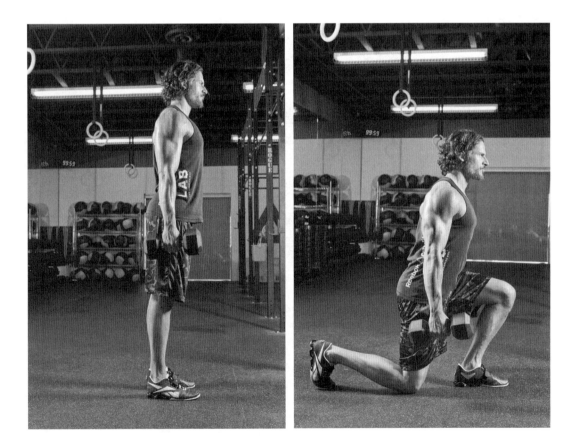

BOX OR BENCH JUMP

1. Stand behind a high box, with your feet positioned in between hip- and shoulder-width apart.

2. Swing your arms back and squat down slightly.

3. Explosively swing your arms forward and jump onto the box. Land lightly, with your feet hip-width apart.

4. Stand tall on top of the box. Carefully step off the box.

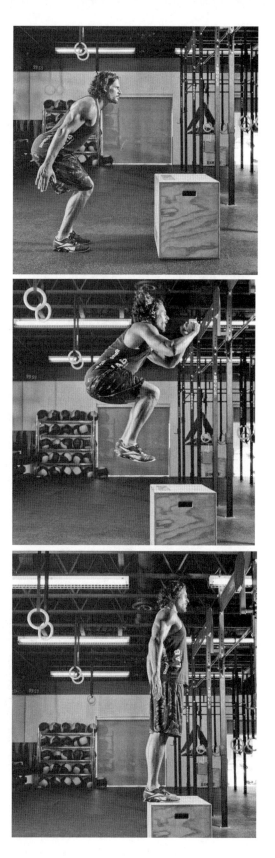

ONE-LEG BENCH BRIDGE

1. Sit on the floor with your left foot on the ground, your right leg bent and elevated, and your upper back resting on a bench.

2. Place your arms out to the sides and push your hips upward, keeping your right leg elevated.

3. Pause, and then slowly lower your body and leg back to the starting position.

4. Complete the prescribed number of reps with your left leg, and then switch legs and do the same number with your right leg.

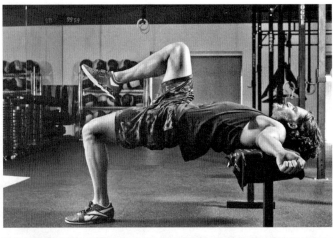

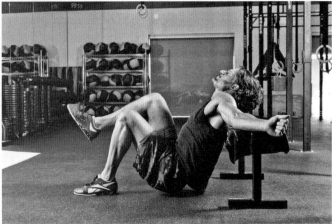

BENCH JUMP-OVER

1. Place your hands on a bench and start in the top position of a push-up. Your body should form a straight line from your shoulders to your ankles. Then, walk your feet to one side of the bench so that your torso is at an angle to the bench. This is your starting position.

2. In one explosive movement, dip your knees and explosively jump laterally toward the other side of the bench while keeping your hands on the bench at all times. Immediately dip your knees and then jump back to the other side.

3. Repeat for the prescribed number of reps.

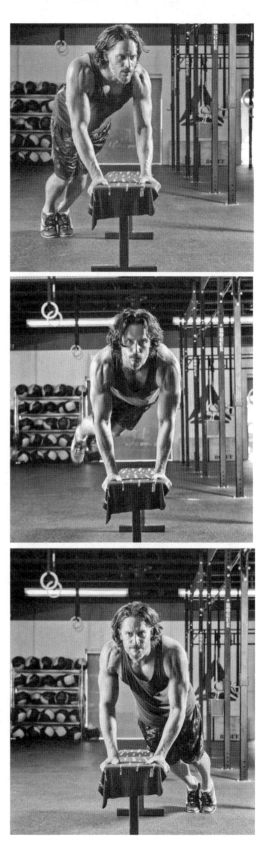

BURPEE

1. Stand with your feet shoulder-width apart and your arms at your sides.

2. Push back your hips, bend your knees, and lower your body as deep as you can into a squat.

3. Place your palms on the floor and then kick your legs backward, so that you're now in a push-up position.

4. Quickly bring back your legs to the squat position and jump up quickly back to the starting position.

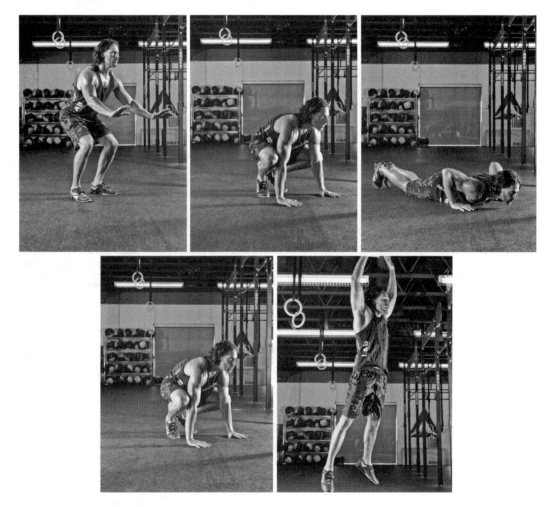

V-BAR TRICEPS EXTENSION

1. Facing the pulley station, grab the V-handle attachment set to a high pulley with an overhand grip.

2. Holding the attachment, bring your elbows to your sides so that your forearms are parallel to the floor. This is the starting position, and from here your elbows shouldn't move.

3. Extend your forearms straight down by contracting the triceps.

4. Hold at lockout with your arms fully extended for one second before returning to the starting position.

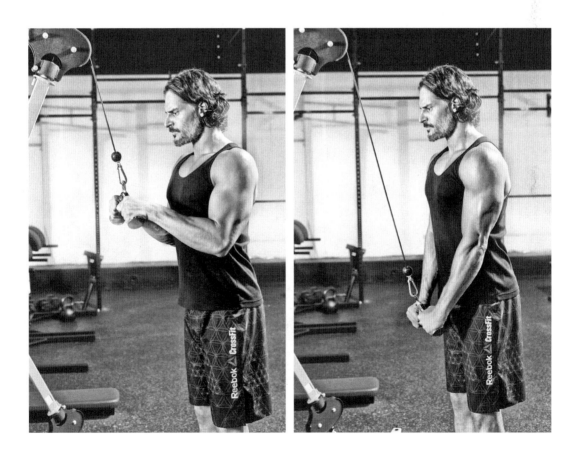

STRAIGHT-BAR TRICEPS EXTENSION

1. Facing the pulley station, grab the straight-bar attachment set to a high pulley with a shoulder-width overhand grip.

2. Holding the attachment, bring your elbows to your sides so that your forearms are parallel to the floor. This is the starting position, and from here your elbows shouldn't move.

3. Extend your forearms straight down by contracting the triceps, rotating the attachment slightly so that your knuckles face the floor at the bottom.

4. Hold at lockout for one second before returning to the starting position.

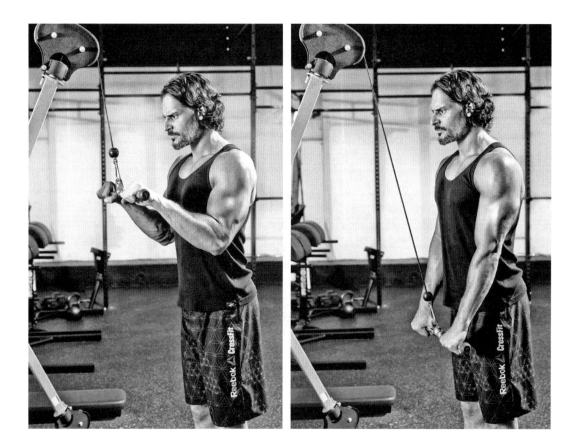

ROPE TRICEPS EXTENSION IN FRONT OF BODY

1. Facing the pulley station, grab the rope attachment set to a high pulley with a thumbs-up grip.

2. Holding the attachment, bring your elbows to your sides so that your forearms are parallel to the floor. This is the starting position, and from here your elbows shouldn't move.

3. Extend your forearms straight down by contracting the triceps, twisting the rope so that your knuckles face the floor at the bottom.

4. Hold at lockout for one second before returning to the starting position.

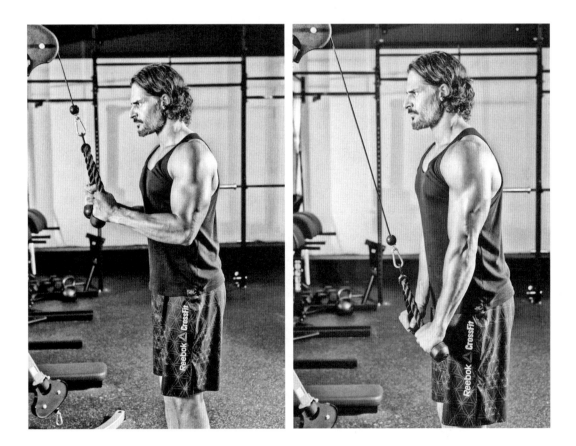

ROPE TRICEPS EXTENSION—OVERHEAD

1. Stand with your back to a high pulley station with a rope attachment.

2. Holding the rope, fully extend your arms overhead and in front of you. This is your starting position.

3. Lower the rope by bending your elbows. Get a good stretch in the triceps and stop when your forearms touch your biceps.

4. Pause for one second in the bottom position and then extend the rope back to the starting position by contracting the triceps. As you press up, twist the ends of the rope so that your knuckles are facing the ceiling at lockout.

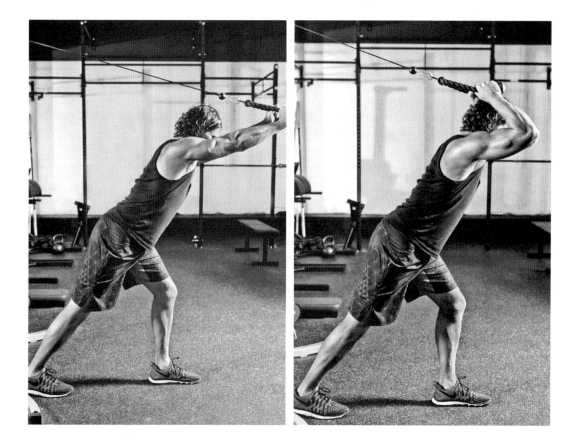

FRENCH PRESS

1. Grab an EZ-curl bar with an overhand grip, sit on the edge of a bench, and position your hands a little less than shoulder-width apart.

2. Keeping your feet flat on the floor, hold the EZ-bar above your head. Without moving your upper arms, lower the bar behind your head.

3. Pause, and then press the weight back to the starting position.

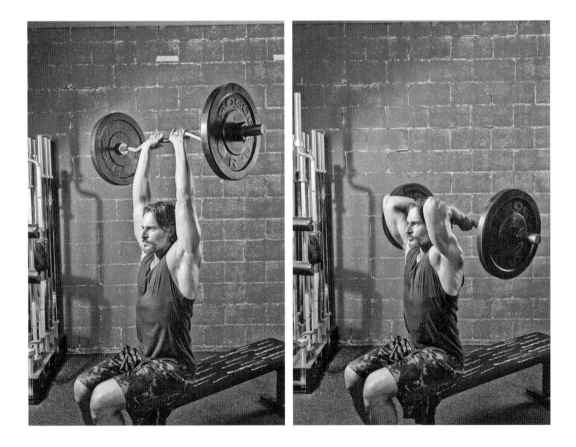

EZ-BAR NOSEBUSTER

1. Grab an EZ-curl bar with an overhand grip, your hands a little less than shoulder-width apart.

2. Keeping your feet flat on the floor, lie faceup on a flat bench and hold the bar with your straight arms over your forehead so that your arms are at an angle. Your arms should be angled back slightly and completely straight.

3. Without moving your upper arms, bend your elbows to lower the bar just past parallel to the floor, keeping elbows as close together as possible.

4. Pause, then lift the weight back to the starting position by straightening your arms.

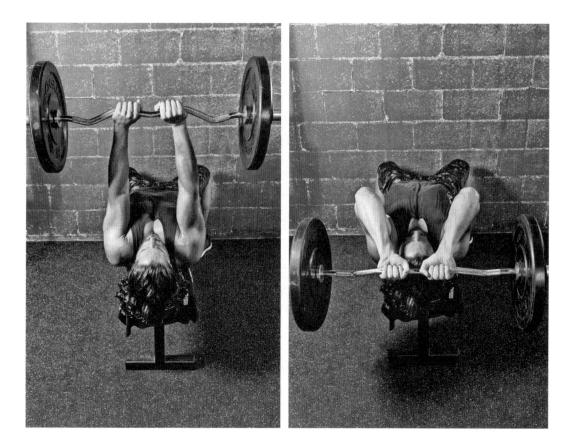

BODY-WEIGHT NOSEBUSTER

1. Set a bar in a rack set to waist height. Assume a push-up position on top of the bar, hands a little closer than shoulder-width apart.

2. Keeping your torso rigid and elbows tucked in, lower your body so that you bend at the elbows and your head goes to the bar. Then straighten your arms and return to the top position.

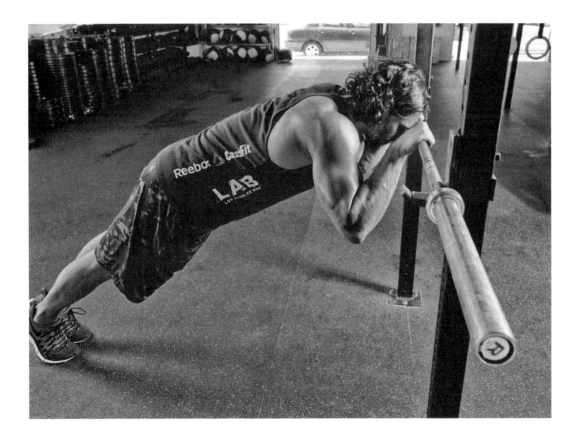

EZ-BAR (OR BARBELL) TRICEPS PRESS WITH NARROW GRIP

1. Grab an EZ-curl bar or a barbell with an overhand, narrow grip, and hold the bar above your sternum with your arms straight.

2. Lower the bar straight down as you tuck your elbows close to your sides.

3. Pause, press the bar back to the starting position, and repeat.

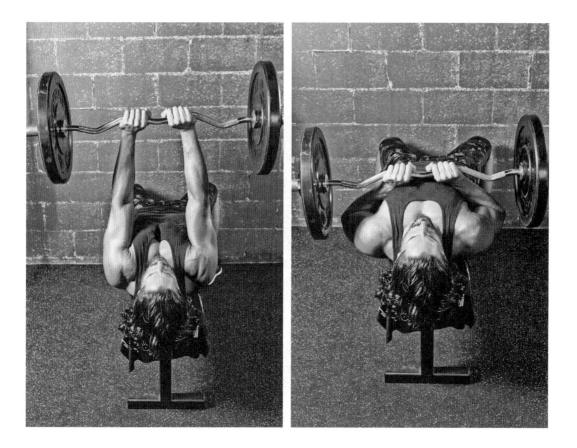

ONE-ARM DUMBBELL LYING TRICEPS EXTENSION

1. Grab one dumbbell and lie faceup on a flat bench. Hold the dumbbell over your head with your arm straight, angled back slightly, your palm facing inward.

2. Without moving your upper arm and keeping your feet flat on the floor, bend your elbow to lower the dumbbell until your forearm is past parallel to the floor.

3. Pause, then lift the weight back to the starting position by straightening your arm. Do all reps, and then switch arms and repeat.

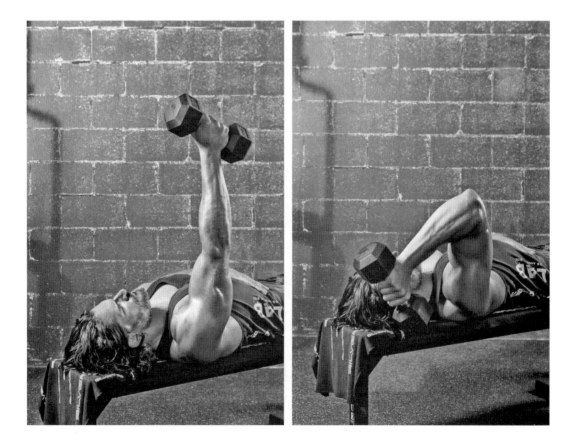

ONE-ARM LYING CROSS-BODY DUMBBELL TRICEPS EXTENSION

1. Grab one dumbbell and lie faceup on a flat bench. Hold the dumbbell over your head with your arm straight, angled back slightly, and rotate your arm so your palm faces forward toward your feet.

2. Without moving your upper arm and keeping your feet flat on the floor, bend one elbow to lower the dumbbell until your forearm is past parallel to the floor and the dumbbell almost touches your opposite shoulder.

3. Pause, then lift the weight back to the starting position by straightening your arm. Do all reps, and then switch arms.

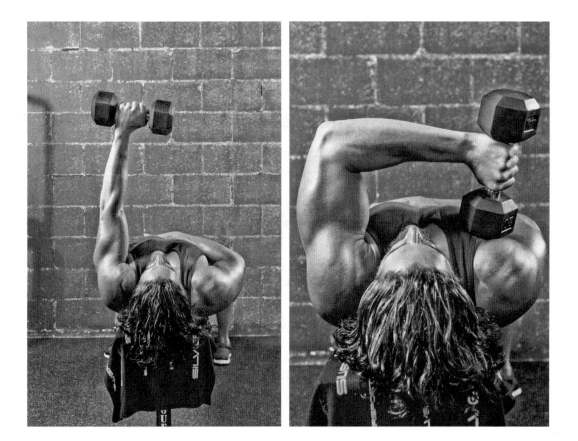

TWO-ARM, ONE-DUMBBELL OVERHEAD TRICEPS EXTENSION

1. Grab a dumbbell and sit with your feet shoulder-width apart. Hold the dumbbell at arm's length above your head, your palms facing up.

2. Without moving your upper arms, lower the dumbbell behind your head.

3. Pause, and then straighten your arms to return the dumbbell to the starting position.

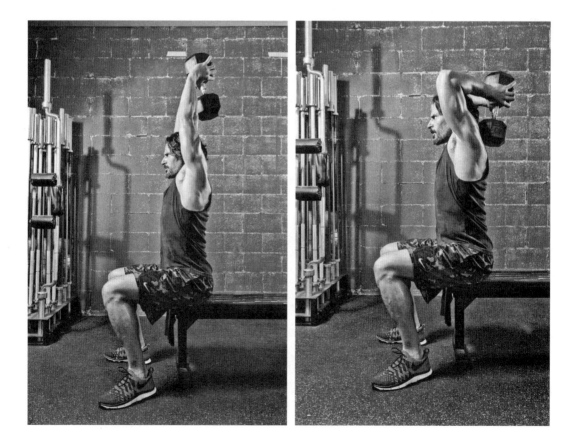

BENCH DIP

1. Sit on the end of a bench or chair with your hands on the edge. Move your feet out in front of you and slide your body forward until your legs are straight and your arms are behind you, supporting your weight. Your arms should be straight, elbows unlocked.

2. Lower your body until your upper arms are parallel to the floor.

3. Pause, then push yourself back up until your arms are straight.

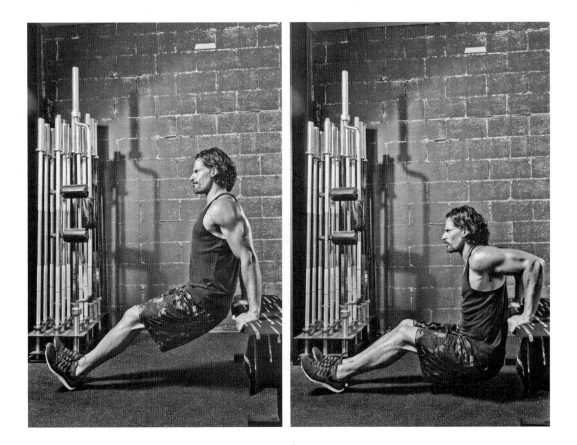

LYING J PRESS

1. Grab a barbell with an overhand, shoulder-width grip, and hold the bar above your sternum with your arms straight.

2. Lower the bar on angle as you tuck your elbows close to your sides so the bar is just above your lower chest.

3. Pause, press the bar back to the starting position, and repeat.

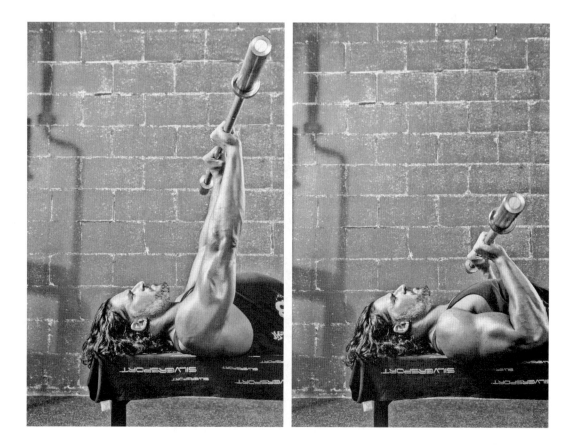

DIAMOND PUSH-UP

1. Assume a push-up position, with your hands touching.

2. Lower your chest to your hands, pause, and push back up.

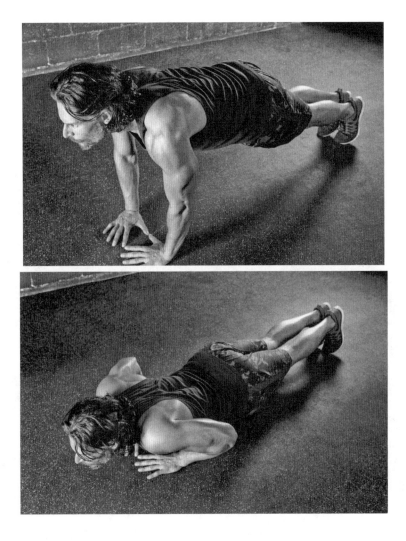

ONE-ARM CABLE TRICEPS EXTENSION

1. Grab the D-handle attachment or the ball at the end of the cable, if it is comfortable in your hand, and stand facing the station.

2. Start with your hand as high as possible without your elbow losing contact with your body and your wrist in a neutral position.

3. Flex the forearm down until you have achieved a lockout position and hold for one second with the arm parallel to the body.

4. Resist the weight as your forearm returns to the starting position.

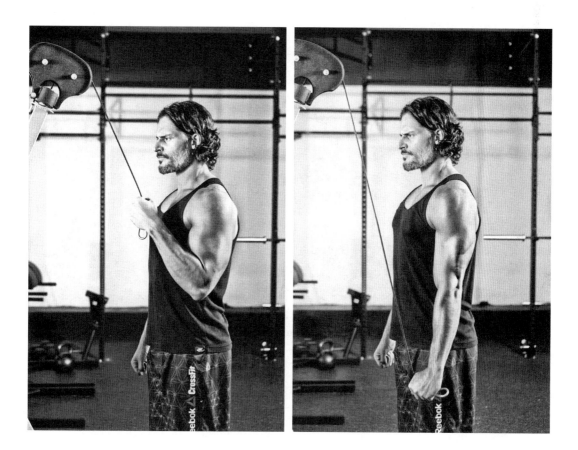

DELTOIDS
STANDING MILITARY PRESS

1. Stand with your feet hip-width apart and hold a barbell in front of your chest, with your hands shoulder-width apart. Your elbows should point downward, and your wrists should be straight.

2. Brace your abs and squeeze your butt. Press the barbell overhead. Lock your arms above your head and stay tall. Do not lean back.

3. Carefully return the weight to the starting position.

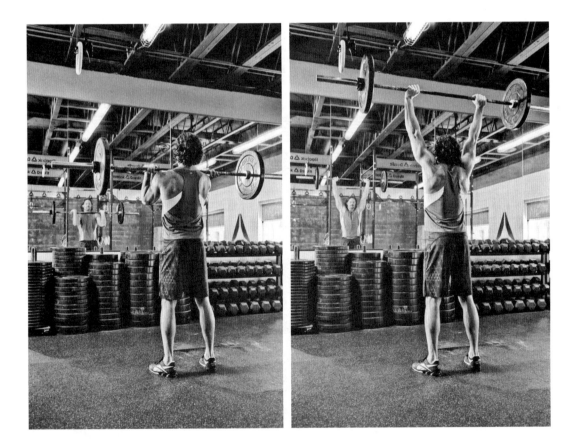

SEATED MILITARY PRESS

1. Grab a barbell using a double-overhand grip so that your hands are slightly wider than shoulder-width apart.

2. Sit on a bench (preferably with an upright back support) and hold the barbell at shoulder height, with your arms bent and elbows by your sides.

3. Gripping the barbell as tight as possible, press it overhead until your elbows are completely locked out.

4. Pause, and then slowly lower the weight back to the starting position.

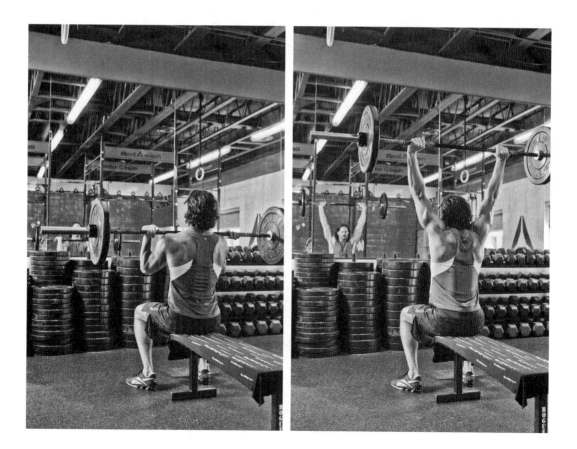

NEUTRAL-GRIP MACHINE OVERHEAD PRESS

1. Sit at an overhead press machine and grab the handles with your arms bent and palms facing each other. Set your feet at shoulder width.

2. Press the handles up until your arms are straight, and then lower back to the starting position.

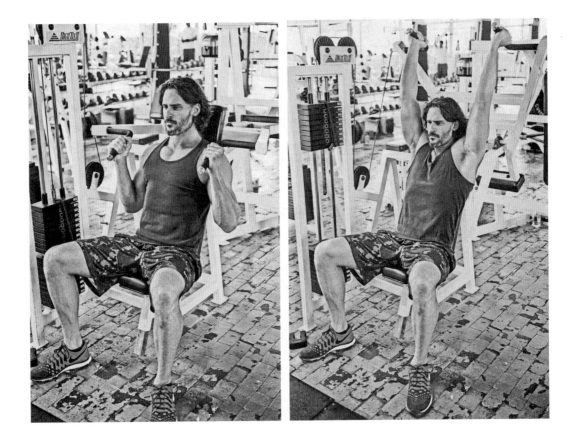

SEATED DUMBBELL OVERHEAD PRESS

1. Sit on a bench (preferably with an upright back support).

2. Grab a set of dumbbells and bring them to shoulder height, with both arms bent and palms facing forward.

3. Gripping the dumbbells as hard as possible, press them overhead until your elbows are completely locked out.

4. Pause, and then slowly lower the weight back to the starting position.

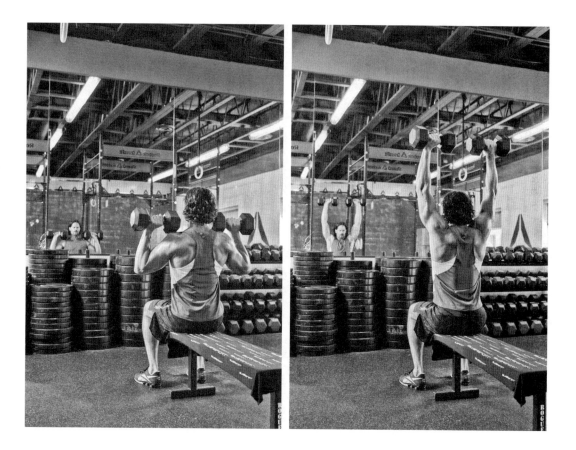

PLATE FRONT RAISE

1. Grab a weight plate on either side, with your thumbs pointing up. Stand tall and allow your arms to hang straight down in front of you.

2. Maintaining a slight bend in your elbows, raise the plate until your arms are just past parallel to the ground.

3. Pause, and then slowly lower the weight back to the starting position.

4. Repeat for the prescribed number of sets and repetitions.

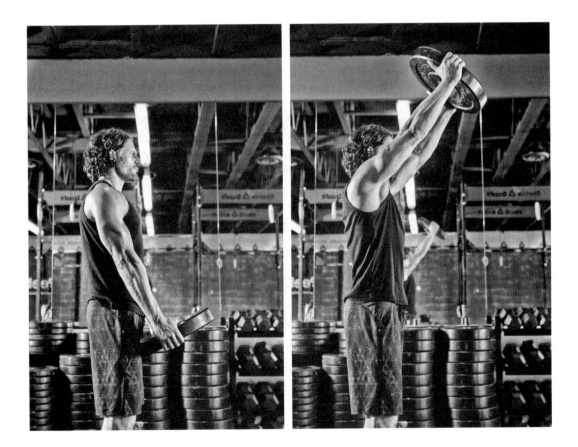

DUMBBELL LATERAL RAISE

1. Grab a pair of dumbbells and let them hang at arm's length in front of you.

2. Stand as tall as you can, with your feet shoulder-width apart. Hold the dumbbells so your palms are facing each other and bend your elbows slightly.

3. Without changing the bend in your elbows, raise your arms straight out to your sides until they're at shoulder level and form a T with your body.

4. Pause for 1 second at the top of the movement, then slowly lower the weights back to the starting position

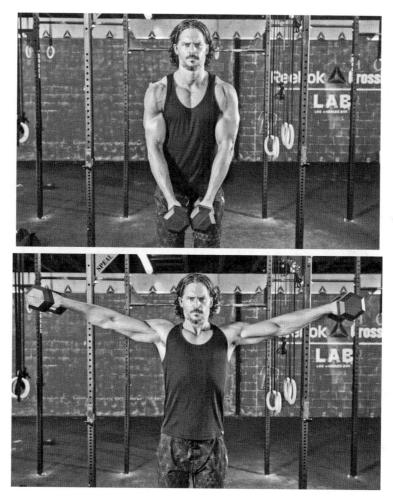

CABLE ONE-ARM LATERAL RAISE

1. Stand in the middle of a dual cable machine, with one weight stack on either side of you. Adjust the handles to the lowest settings.

2. Grab the right handle with your left hand. Stand tall and keep your feet shoulder-width apart.

3. Maintaining a slight bend in the elbow, lift your arm straight out to the side until it is parallel to the ground.

4. Pause, and then slowly return the weight back to the starting position.

5. Repeat for the prescribed number of repetitions, then switch arms.

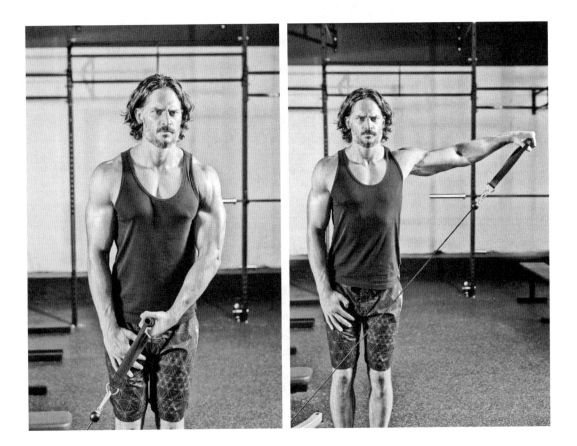

CABLE ONE-ARM BENT-OVER REAR-DELTOID RAISE

1. Stand in the middle of a dual cable machine, with one weight stack on either side of you. Adjust the handles to the lowest settings.

2. Grab the right handle with your left hand. Keeping your spine flat, push your butt backward and bend your torso over until your chest is nearly parallel to the ground.

3. Maintaining a slight bend in the elbows, hold your arm straight out to the side until it's parallel to the ground.

4. Pause, and then slowly return the weight back to the starting position.

5. Repeat for the prescribed number of repetitions and then switch arms.

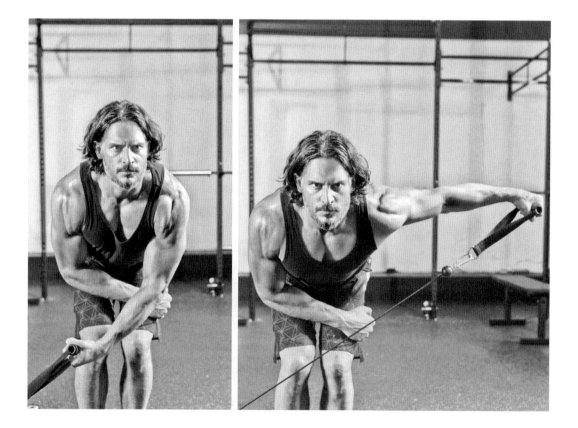

DUMBBELL ROTATING LATERAL RAISE

1. Grab a pair of dumbbells and let them hang at arm's length next to your sides with your palms facing forward. Curl the dumbbells so that your elbows are bent to 90 degrees. Stand as tall as you can, with your feet shoulder-width apart.

2. Without changing the bend in your elbows, raise your arms straight out to your sides as you rotate your palms so that they face the floor. Stop the movement once your elbows are at shoulder level and form a T with your body.

3. Pause for a second at the top of the movement, then slowly lower the weights back to the starting position.

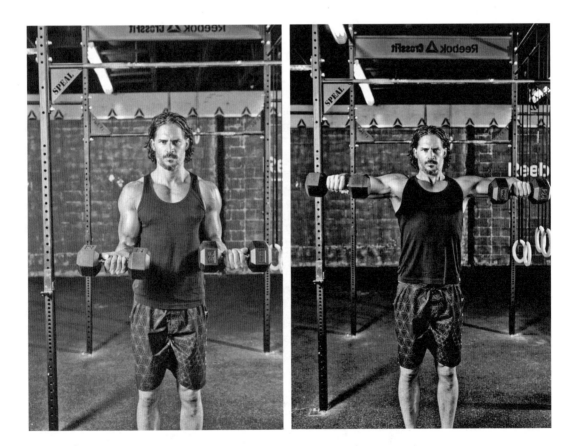

DUMBBELL FRONT RAISE

1. Stand tall with your feet hip-width apart. Hold a dumbbell in each hand in front of your thighs. Your palms should face toward you.

2. Raise your arms up in front of you. Pause once the dumbbells reach shoulder height.

3. Return the weights to the starting position.

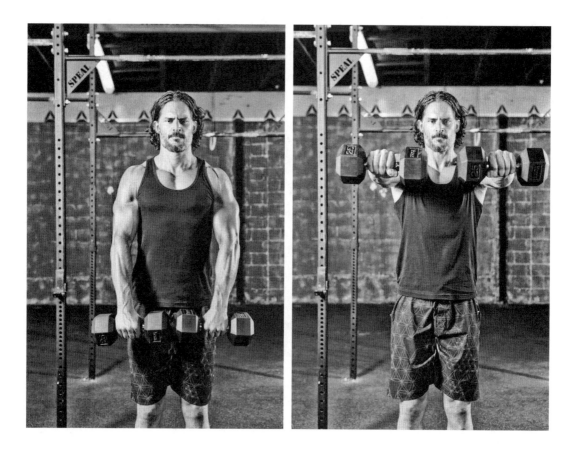

ROPE FRONT RAISE

1. Stand tall in front of and facing away from an adjustable cable machine. Between your legs, hold the handle of a rope attachment positioned to the low setting.

2. Keep your chest up and shoulders back. Lift your arms in front of you, keeping your elbows straight. Pause once your arms reach shoulder height.

3. Return the weight to the beginning position.

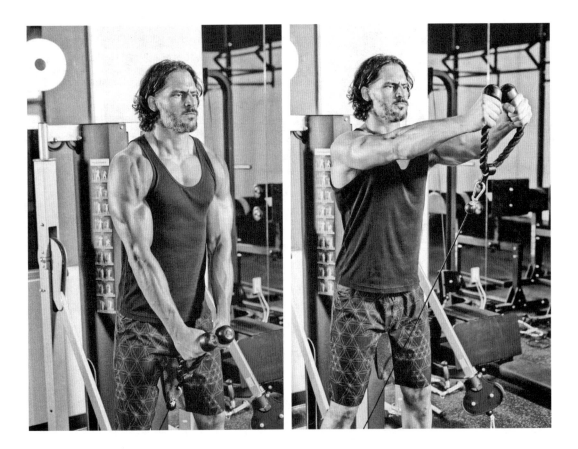

DUMBBELL REAR-DELTOID RAISE

1. Grab a set of dumbbells and stand up with your arms completely straight and your palms facing each other.

2. Keeping your spine flat, push your butt backward toward the wall behind you, slightly bend your knees, and bend your torso until your upper body is nearly parallel to the ground. Your arms should be hanging beneath your chest.

3. Maintaining a slight bend in your elbows, raise your arms up and out to the sides of your body until they are in line with your shoulders.

4. Pause, and then slowly lower the weights back to the starting position.

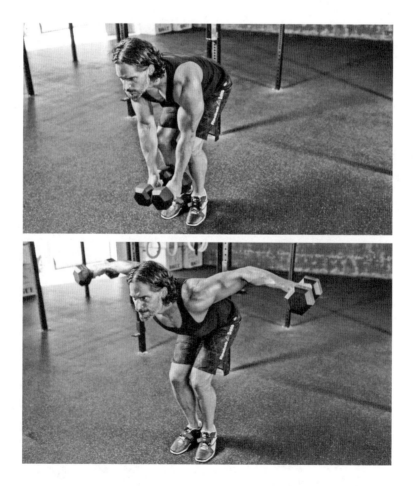

DUMBBELL FRONT RAISE AND LATERAL RAISE

1. Stand tall with your feet hip-width apart. Hold a dumbbell in each hand in front of your thighs. Your palms should face toward you. Raise your arms in front of you. Pause once the dumbbells reach shoulder height. Return the weights to the starting position.

2. Raise your arms to the side. Pause once the dumbbells reach shoulder height. Return the weights to the starting position. That's one rep.

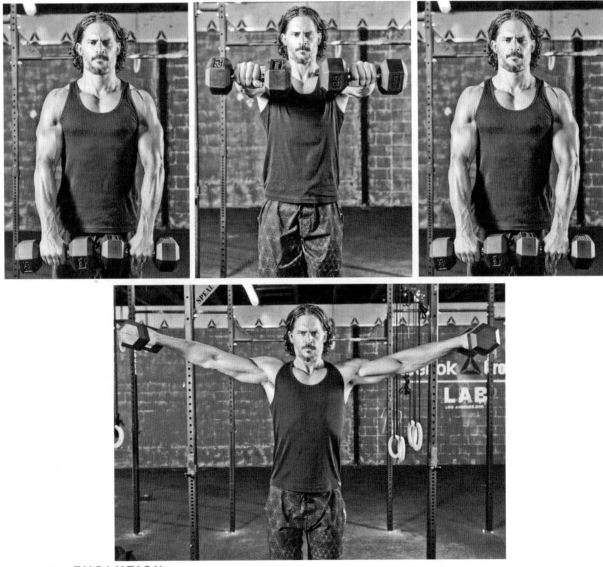

BARBELL UPRIGHT ROW

1. Grab a barbell with an overhand grip, your hands about shoulder-width apart.

2. Keeping the bar as close to your body as possible, pull the bar up toward your chest.

3. Your elbows should remain flared out during the movement.

4. When the bar is at your chest level (and not your chin), pause for 1 to 2 seconds, and then lower the bar back to the starting position.

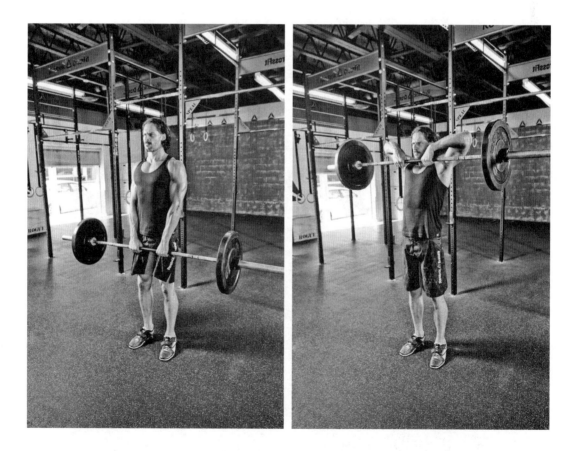

SEATED ARNOLD PRESS

1. Sit on a bench (preferably with a back support), so that your torso is upright.

2. Grab a set of dumbbells and bring them to shoulder height, with both arms bent and palms facing forward.

3. Gripping the dumbbells as tight as possible, press them overhead until your elbows are completely locked out.

4. Pause, and then slowly lower the weight until your elbows are bent to 90 degrees.

5. Rotate your forearms so that your palms are pointing toward your face and the inner plates of the dumbbells lightly touch each other.

6. Pause, and then return to the starting position.

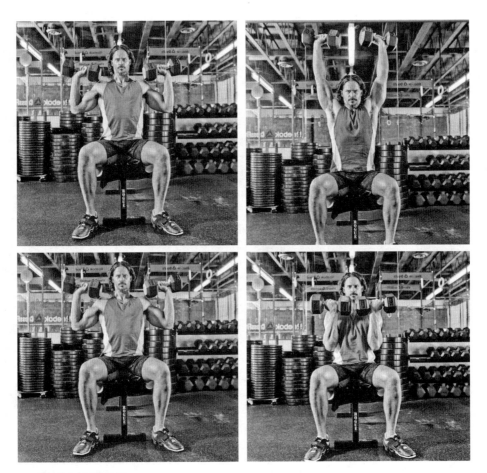

SEATED REAR-DELTOID BENT-OVER DUMBBELL REVERSE FLYE

1. Grab a pair of dumbbells, sit on the edge of a bench, and hold the weights at arm's length, your palms facing each other.

2. Keeping your lower back naturally arched, bend at your hips and slightly lower your torso toward the floor. Without moving your torso or changing the bend in your elbows, raise your arms straight out to your sides until they're in line with your body.

3. Pause, then slowly return to the starting position.

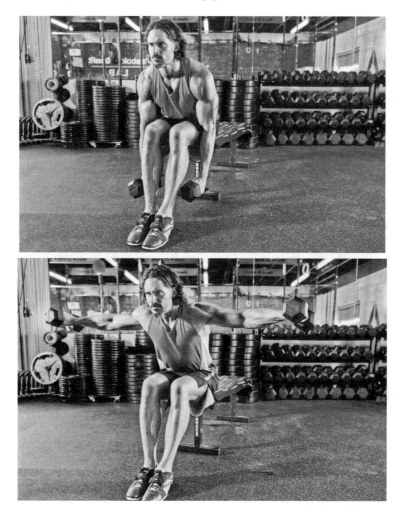

CABLE TWO-ARM REVERSE FLYE

1. Stand in the middle of a dual cable machine, with one weight stack on either side of you. Adjust the handles to be even with your chest, grab the right handle with your left hand and the left handle with your right hand. Keep an upright posture with your spine flat.

2. Maintaining a slight bend in the elbows, move your arms straight out to the side, keeping the arms parallel to the ground until they are straight out from your body, making the letter T.

3. Pause, then slowly return the weight back to the starting position.

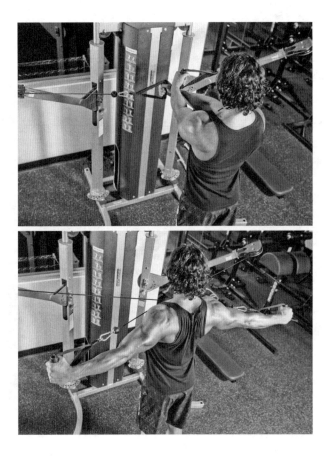

STANDING BARBELL CURL

1. Grab a barbell with an underhand grip and let it hang at arm's length, with your palms facing forward.

2. Without moving your upper arms, bend your elbows and curl the barbell as close to your shoulders as you can.

3. Pause, and then lower the barbell back to the starting position.

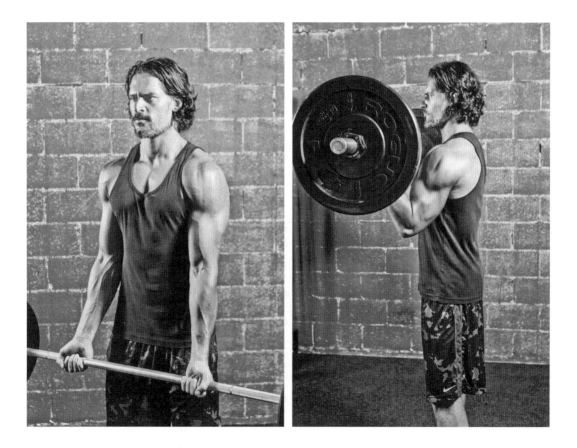

EZ-BAR CURL WITH NARROW GRIP

1. Grab an EZ-curl bar with an underhand, narrow grip. The bar should hang at arm's length in front of your waist.

2. Without moving your upper arms, bend your elbows and curl the bar as close to your shoulders as you can.

3. Pause, and then lower the weight back to the starting position.

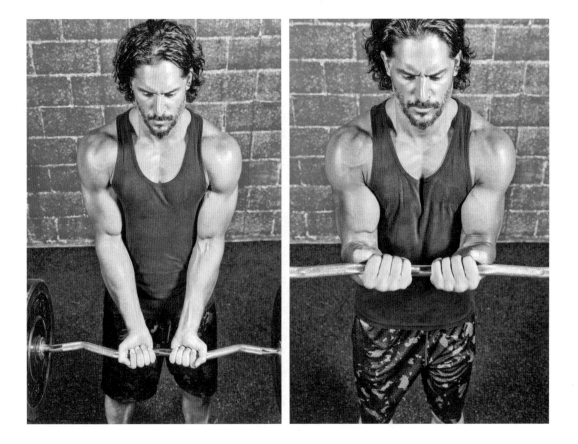

EZ-BAR CURL WITH OUTSIDE GRIP

1. Grab an EZ-curl bar with an underhand, shoulder-width grip. The bar should hang at arm's length in front of your waist.

2. Without moving your upper arms, bend your elbows and curl the bar as close to your shoulders as you can.

3. Pause, and then lower the weight back to the starting position.

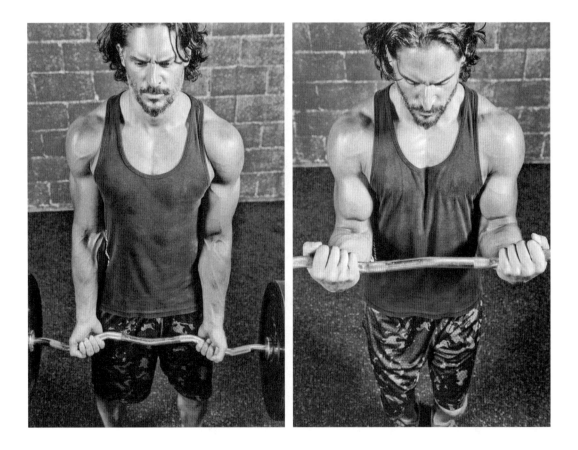

PREACHER CURL

1. Rest your upper arms on the sloping pad of a preacher bench and hold the bar in front of you, with your elbows bent about 5 degrees and your hands about 6 inches apart.

2. Without moving your upper arms and keeping them on the pad, bend your elbows and curl the bar toward your shoulders.

3. Pause, and then slowly lower the weight back to the starting position.

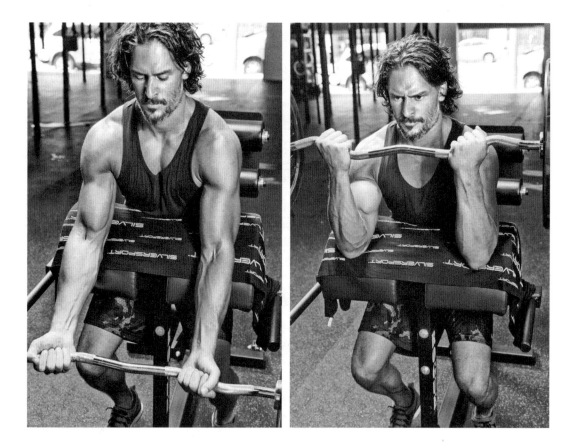

PREACHER CURL PULSE

1. Rest your upper arms on the sloping pad of a preacher bench and hold the bar in front of you, your elbows bent about 5 degrees and your hands about 6 inches apart.

2. Without moving your upper arms and keeping them on the pad, bend your elbows and curl the bar toward your shoulders. When you curl the weight as high as you can, perform mini "pulsing" reps where you squeeze your biceps at the peak.

3. Pause, then slowly lower the weight back to the starting position.

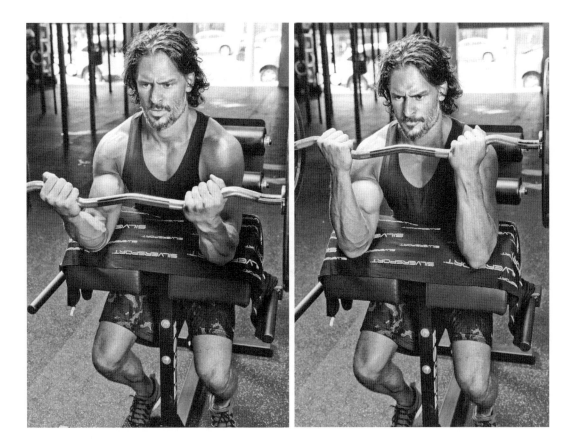

SEATED DUMBBELL TWO-ARM CURL

1. Sit on a bench, grab a pair of dumbbells, and let them hang at arm's length next to your sides, with your palms facing forward.

2. Without moving your upper arms, bend your elbows and curl the dumbbells as close to your shoulders as you can.

3. Pause, and then lower the weights back to the starting position.

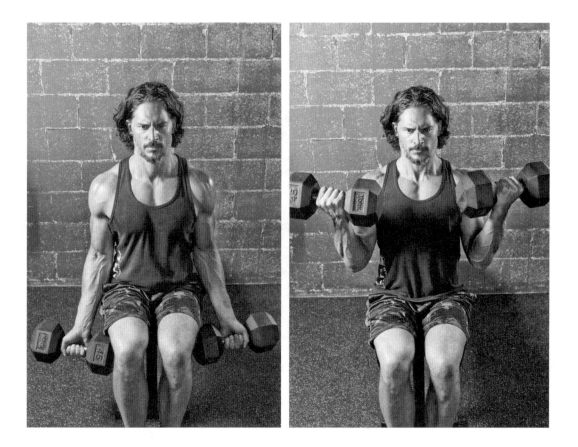

DUMBBELL HAMMER CURL

1. Grab a set of dumbbells with a neutral grip so that your palms are facing each other; stand tall with your feet shoulder-width apart.

2. While bracing your core, curl the dumbbells all the way up to shoulder height while keeping your palms facing each other.

3. Pause at the top and squeeze your biceps, and then lower the weights back down to the starting position.

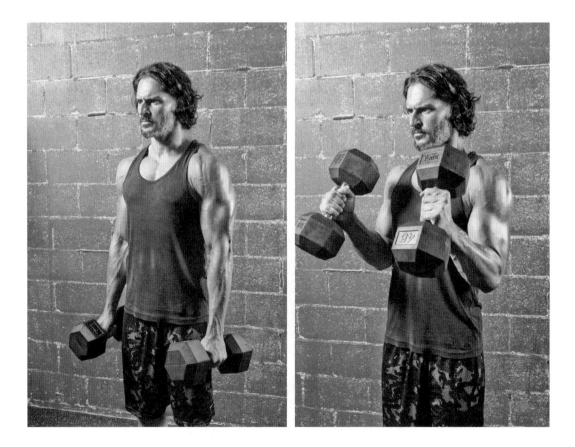

ROPE HAMMER CURL

1. Grab a rope attachment with a neutral grip—your palms facing each other—and let it hang at arm's length.

2. Without moving your upper arms, bend your elbows and curl the rope as close to your shoulders as you can.

3. Pause, and then lower the bar back to the starting position.

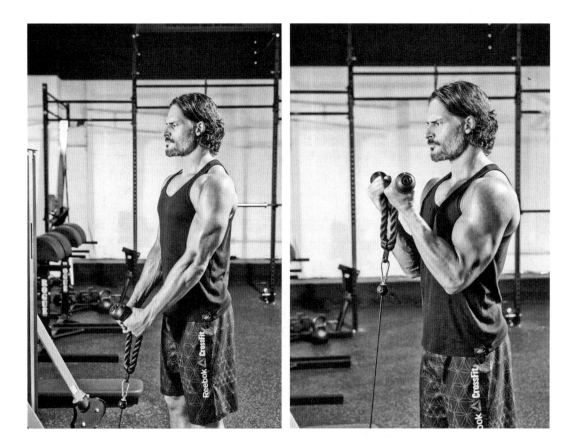

TRIPLE DUMBBELL CURL

1. With arms held out straight in front of you, parallel to the ground, do alternating curls for the specified number of reps, holding the weight extended from the body when not curling.

2. With arms at sides, do traditional curls with both arms moving at the same time for the same number of reps.

3. Sit back on an incline bench and have your arms hang straight down. Do curls with both arms together for the same number of reps, focusing on trying to curl your pinky finger into your armpit without moving the angle of the upper arm (don't swing).

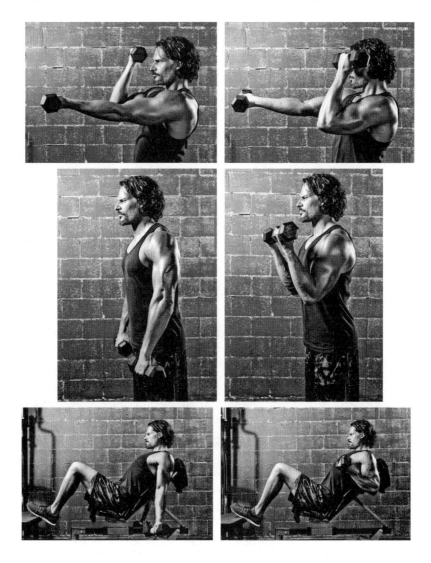

STRAIGHT-BAR CABLE CURL

1. Grab a straight-bar cable attachment with an underhand grip and let it hang at arm's length, with your palms facing forward.

2. Without moving your upper arms, bend your elbows and curl the bar as close to your shoulders as you can.

3. Pause, and then lower the bar back to the starting position.

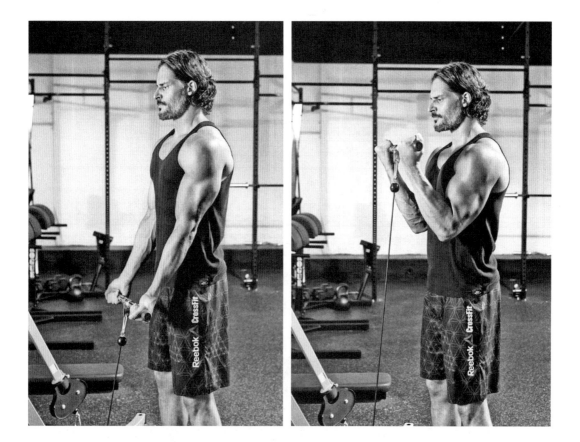

DUMBBELL ALTERNATING CURL

1. Stand with your feet shoulder-width apart; hold a dumbbell in each hand with your palms facing forward.

2. Curl the right dumbbell toward the right shoulder. The other dumbbell should remain at your left side. Try to minimize moving the elbow (shoulder flexion) or cheating with the lower back.

3. Hold at the top for 1 second and return to the starting position, and then repeat the movement using the left dumbbell.

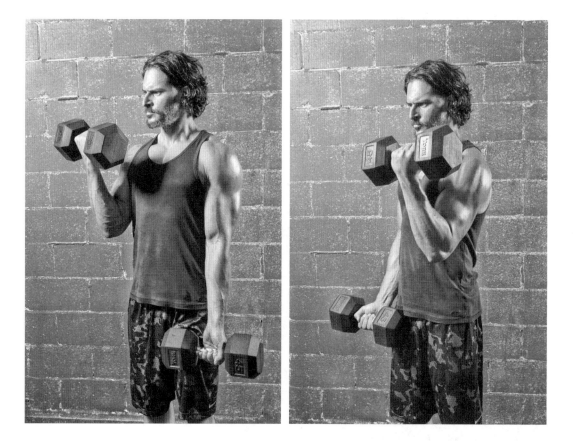

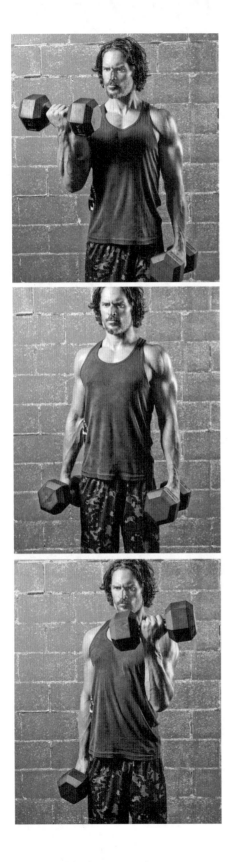

DUMBBELL ALTERNATING CURL WITH TWIST

1. Stand with your feet shoulder-width apart; hold a dumbbell in each hand with an overhand grip and your palms facing your sides.

2. Curl the right dumbbell toward the right shoulder. The other dumbbell should remain at your left side. Try to minimize moving the elbow (shoulder flexion) or cheating with the lower back.

3. As you curl the weight up, twist the pinky finger of the working arm toward the ceiling. This intensifies the contraction in the biceps.

4. Hold at the top for 1 second and return to the starting position, and then repeat the movement using the left dumbbell.

REVERSE CURL

1. Grasp a barbell with an overhand, palms-down grip, with your hands shoulder-width apart.

2. Allow your arms to hang straight down without locking your elbows; keep your shoulders pulled back. Curl the bar toward your shoulders.

3. At the top, hold the weight for a moment before lowering it under control.

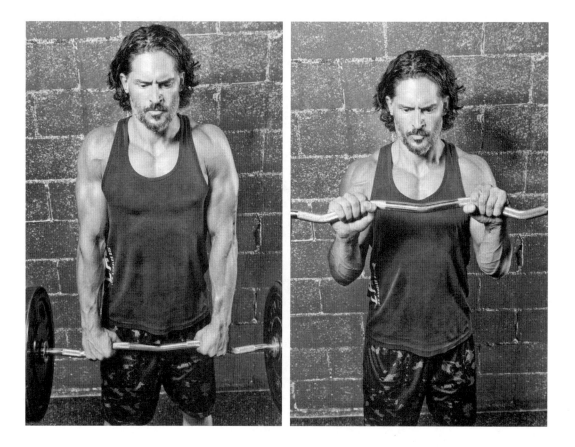

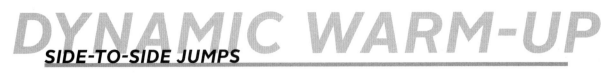

SIDE-TO-SIDE JUMPS

1. Find a line on the floor. It can be a seam between floorboards or mats, a piece of tape, your jump rope or a towel—anything handy.

2. Place both feet together on one side of the line. Hop sideways over the line back and forth for 30 seconds without stopping. Try to rebound quickly off of the floor and always jump off of and land both feet at the same time.

FRONT-TO-BACK JUMPS

1. Find a line on the floor. It can be a seam between floorboards or mats, a piece of tape, your jump rope or a towel—anything handy.

2. Place both feet together on one side of the line. Hop forward and backwards over the line for 30 seconds without stopping. Try not to hit the line, especially on the way back.

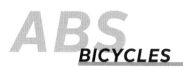

BICYCLES

1. Lie flat on the floor with your hands behind your ears. Raise your legs about 6 inches off the floor and bring your shoulders up, so that your arms are in a wide V.

2. Next, use your abs to drive your right elbow toward your left knee, release, and then drive your left elbow toward your right knee. Continue alternating sides.

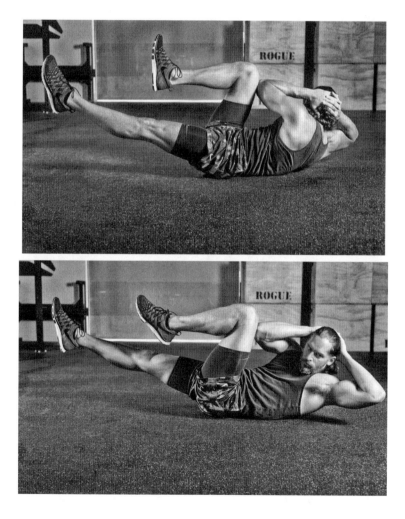

CRUNCH

1. Lie on your back with your knees bent. Place your fingers lightly behind your ears—but don't pull on your neck.

2. Slowly curl your torso toward your knees, bringing your shoulders 4 to 6 inches off the floor. Hold for a few seconds with your lower back pressed to the floor.

3. Slowly lower your body back to the starting position.

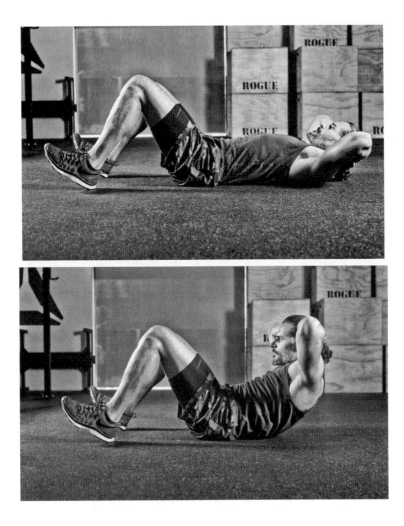

HANGING LEG RAISE

1. Grip a bar with your hands spaced a little more than shoulder-width apart. Your legs should hang straight down.

2. Curl your trunk upwards by rotating your pelvis towards your body, then slowly raise your knees towards your chest as high as you can. Try not to arch your back.

3. Now slowly lower your knees until your legs are back in the starting position.

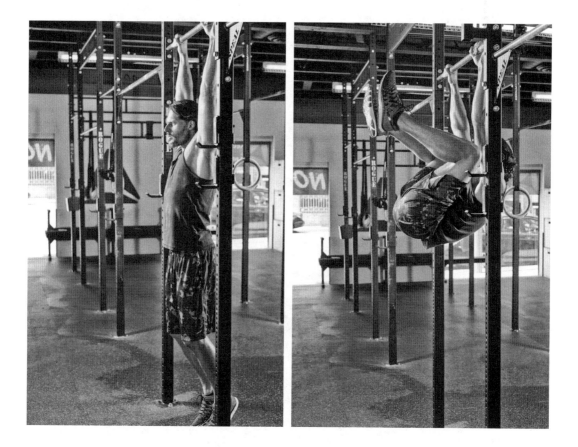

HIP-UPS

1. Lie faceup on a bench. Grab the bench next to your head and straighten your legs while keeping your lower back firmly pressed into the bench.

2. Start by slowly bringing your knees up, rolling the hips off the bench until your knees touch your elbows.

3. Then slowly lower your hips back onto the bench, feeling each vertebra touch in succession.

4. When the hips are on the bench, slowly extend the feet out until the legs are straight.

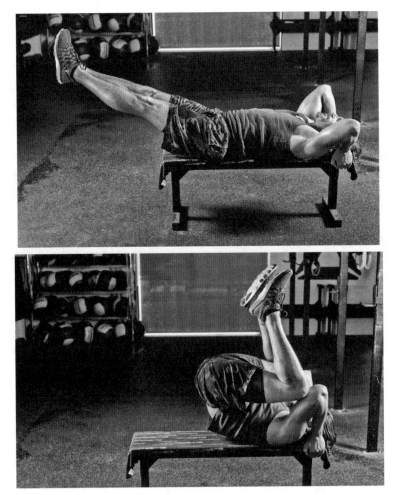

REVERSE BICYCLE

1. Start in the same position as a bicycle. Begin pedaling your feet as if you were pedaling a giant bicycle backward.

2. While keeping the hands behind the head and shoulder blades off of the ground twist the upper body as one piece to touch the left elbow to the right knee as it comes around, then the right elbow to the left knee, and so on.

3. Note: The tempo of this exercise is slow, with a full extension of the legs.

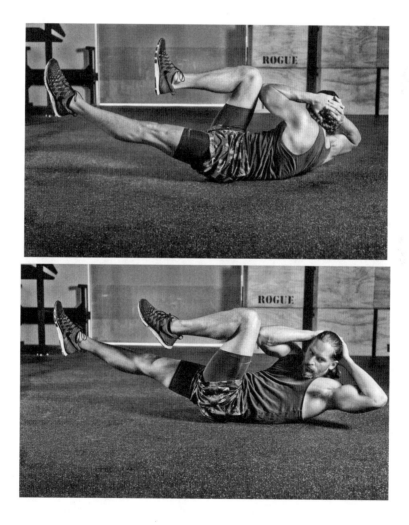

MOUNTAIN CLIMBER

1. Assume a push-up position with your hands slightly wider than your shoulders. Your body should form a straight line from your ankles to your head.

2. Brace your abdominals—as if you were about to be punched in the gut—and maintain that contraction for the duration of this exercise. Lift your right foot off the floor and raise your knee as close to your chest as you can. Don't change your lower-back posture as you lift your knee.

3. Touch the floor with your right foot, then return to the starting position. Repeat with your left leg.

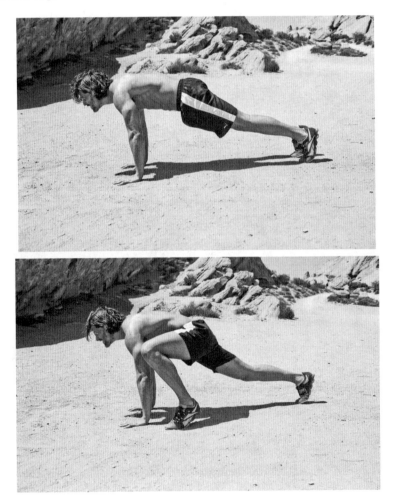

TOES TO BAR

1. Hang from a pull-up bar with your hands about shoulder-width apart and keep your arms and legs as straight as possible.

2. Swing your legs forward and touch your feet to the bar above your head, and then fully extend your legs and feet back down to the ground. Each touch of your feet to the bar counts as one rep.

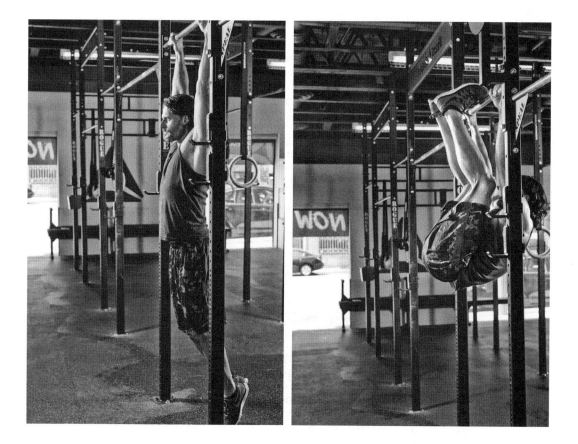

ACKNOWLEDGMENTS

Thank you to . . . the number one fitness authority on the planet, Adam Bornstein, without whom none of this would have been possible.

Thank you, Simon Green and CAA. Jeremie Ruby-Strauss, Emilia Pisani, Jen Bergstrom, and the team at Simon & Schuster's Gallery Books.

Colleen Schlegel at Artist Management. Lisa Perkins at Fifteen Minutes. The "B&R West Side Guys." My bros Rich, Robbie, and Geoff, aka "the 'Scoes cheat-meal gang."

The number one fitness photographer in the world, Patrik Giardino. Shawn Perine and *Muscle & Fitness* magazine. Dan Jones. *Men's Health* magazines worldwide. *Muscle & Body* magazine. Brantt Myhres. David Paul. Gordon Alatorre and GLA Masonry. Rodolfo Martinez. Jo Jo Odyssey. Daniel Ketchell. Jonathan Kundly. Don Swayze, for sharing his inspiring story. Bridget, for all of her love and support and patience and home cooking! My brother and best friend, Nick. My father, for teaching me discipline and to *never* accept anything less than my best. My mother, for feeding me nothing but organic food growing up, for sneaking me into the gym with her for years, and always being my biggest fan.

My mentor, Dr. Jim "Moon Dog" Mooney, for laying the immovable foundation I would always be able to return to, no matter how far away from it I ever got. The icon Arnold Schwarzenegger, for inspiring a generation of men to become stronger and more productive and for being my friend. The best trainer in the world . . . my friend and personal "Dr. Frankenstein," Ron Mathews at Reebok CrossFit LAB, L.A., for changing my life and helping me finally slay the dragon that had been chasing me for as far back as I can remember: my potential.

And to all of the lifting partners, in all of those gyms, in all of those cities, over all of those years, all over the world . . . this is for you.